Core
Clinical
Cases in
Psychiatry

Second edition

2

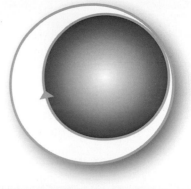

Core
Clinical
Cases in

Psychiatry

A problem-solving approach

Second edition

Tom Clark MB ChB LLM MRCPsych
Consultant Forensic Psychiatrist and Honorary Senior
Clinical Lecturer in Forensic Psychiatry, Birmingham
and Solihull Mental Health NHS Foundation Trust,
Birmingham, UK

Ed Day BA BM BCh DM MRCPsych
Senior Lecturer in Addiction Psychiatry, School of Clinical
and Experimental Medicine, University of Birmingham,
Department of Psychiatry, Edgbaston, UK

Emma C. Fergusson MA BM BCh DCH
MRCPsych
Consultant Child and Adolescent Psychiatrist, South
Oxfordshire CAMHS, UK

Core Clinical Cases series edited by

Janesh K. Gupta MSc, MD FRCOG
Professor in Obstetrics and Gynaecology, University
of Birmingham, Birmingham Women's Hospital,
Birmingham, UK

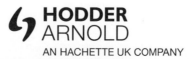
HODDER
ARNOLD
AN HACHETTE UK COMPANY

First published in Great Britain in 2005 by Arnold,
This second edition published in 2011 by Hodder Arnold, an imprint of Hodder Education, a
division of Hachette UK, 338 Euston Road, London NW1 3BH

http://www.hodderarnold.com

Whilst the advice and information in this book are believed to be true and accurate at the date
of going to press, neither the author[s] nor the publisher can accept any legal responsibility or
liability for any errors or omissions that may be made. In particular (but without limiting the
generality of the preceding disclaimer) every effort has been made to check drug dosages;
however it is still possible that errors have been missed. Furthermore, dosage schedules are
constantly being revised and new side effects recognized. For these reasons the reader is strongly
urged to consult the drug companies' printed instructions before administering any of the drugs
recommended in this book.

British Library Cataloguing in Publication Data
A catalogue record for this book is available from the British Library

Library of Congress Cataloging-in-Publication Data
A catalog record for this book is available from the Library of Congress

ISBN-13: 978 1 444 12287 9
1 2 3 4 5 6 7 8 9 10

Commissioning Editor: Joanna Koster
Project Editor: Stephen Clausard
Production Controller: Jonathan Williams
Cover Design: Amina Dudhia
Index: Merrall-Ross International Ltd

Typeset in 9 on 11pt Frutiger by Phoenix Photosetting, Chatham, Kent
Printed in India

What do you think about this book? Or any other Hodder Arnold title?
Please visit our website: www.hodderarnold.com

Contents

Series preface

'A history lesson'

Between about 1916 and 1927 a puzzling illness appeared and swept around the world. Dr von Economo first described encephalitis lethargica (EL), which simply meant 'inflammation of the brain that makes you tired'. Younger people, especially women, seemed to be more vulnerable but the disease affected people of all ages. People with EL developed a 'sleep disorder', fever, headache and weakness, which led to a prolonged state of unconsciousness. The EL epidemic occurred during the same time period as the 1918 influenza pandemic, and the two outbreaks have been linked ever since in the medical literature. Some confused it with the epidemic of Spanish flu at that time while others blamed weapons used in World War I.

Encephalitis lethargica (EL) was dramatized by the film *Awakenings* (book written by Oliver Sacks, an eminent neurologist from New York), starring Robin Williams and Robert De Niro. Professor Sacks treated his patients with L-dopa, which temporarily awoke his patients, giving rise to the belief that the condition was related to Parkinson's disease.

Since the 1916–1927 epidemic, only sporadic cases have been described. Pathological studies have revealed an encephalitis of the midbrain and basal ganglia, with lymphocyte (predominantly plasma cell) infiltration. Recent examination of archived EL brain material has failed to demonstrate influenza RNA, adding to the evidence that EL was not an invasive influenza encephalitis. Further investigations found no evidence of viral encephalitis or other recognized causes of rapid-onset parkinsonism. Magnetic resonance imaging (MRI) of the brain was normal in 60 per cent but showed inflammatory changes localized to the deep grey matter in 40 per cent of patients.

As late as the end of the 20th century, it seemed that the possible answers lay in the clinical presentation of the patients in the 1916–1927 epidemic. It had been noted by the clinicians at that time that the central nervous system (CNS) disorder had presented with pharyngitis. This led to the possibility of a post-infectious autoimmune CNS disorder similar to Sydenham's chorea, in which group A beta-haemolytic streptococcal antibodies cross-react with the basal ganglia and result in abnormal behaviour and involuntary movements. Anti-streptolysin-O titres have subsequently been found to be elevated in the majority of these patients. It seemed possible that autoimmune antibodies may cause remitting parkinsonian signs subsequent to streptococcal tonsillitis as part of the spectrum of post-streptococcal CNS disease.

Could it be that the 80-year mystery of EL has been solved relying on the patient's clinical history of presentation, rather than focusing on expensive investigations? More research in this area will give us the definitive answer. This scenario is not dissimilar to the controversy about the idea that streptococcal infections were aetiologically related to rheumatic fever.

With this example of a truly fascinating history lesson, we hope that you will endeavour to use the patient's clinical history as your most powerful diagnostic tool to make the correct diagnosis. If you do you are likely to be right between 80 and 90 per cent of the time. This is the basis of the Core Clinical Cases series, which will make you systematically explore clinical problems through the clinical history of presentation, followed by examination and then the performance of appropriate investigations. Never break those rules!

Janesh Gupta

2005

Preface

This book aims to present undergraduate medical students with clinical case scenarios that are common in psychiatric practice, and take them through a process of assessment and diagnosis, identifying likely aetiological factors, and considering appropriate treatment options. It has been informed by changes in undergraduate medical education at a national level that are increasingly impacting on the way in which clinical skills are evaluated.

The process of clinical assessment is a little different in psychiatry from other branches of medicine. In psychiatry, all diagnoses are syndromal. Diagnosis depends on the doctor being able to understand clearly a patient's subjective experience, to categorize those experiences in psychopathological terms, and then to recognize those collections of symptoms which go to form recognized syndromes. Physical investigations remain important in psychiatry, but not usually to confirm a diagnosis. Rather, they may be used to exclude physical diagnoses or to support pharmacological treatment. Therefore, for each case in the book, with the exception of Chapter 4 in the Clinical cases section, the first question asks for a differential diagnosis and the second question considers the clinical features which may help to confirm this.

Psychiatric treatment may be diagnosis-specific, for example, antidepressant treatment for a depressive episode. However, in many cases the most appropriate forms of treatment are determined by other factors which are considered to have contributed to the illness. So, a patient with schizophrenia is likely to require treatment with an antipsychotic drug, but other treatments may depend on whether their psychosis has been precipitated by substance misuse, by high expressed emotion in the family, or by poor compliance with maintenance antipsychotic medication. Therefore, as well as making a diagnosis it is necessary to consider aetiological factors, which may represent targets for therapeutic intervention. Question 3 of the Clinical cases section relates to aetiology. This book uses the following terms:

- **Predisposing factors**: These are things which lead to an individual having an increased likelihood of developing a particular illness. Often, they are epidemiologically observed associations.
- **Precipitating factors**: These are factors which have contributed to causing an individual to develop an illness at a particular time.
- **Maintaining factors**: These are factors which may be preventing a patient from recovering, or may be reducing the effectiveness of treatment. Often, there is some overlap between maintaining factors and precipitating factors.

Issues related to culture and diversity are also particularly important in psychiatric assessment and treatment. The presentation of mental illness often reflects cultural beliefs and customs, and the acceptability of certain treatment modalities may also be affected by culturally determined characteristics.

The fourth question relating to each case discusses treatment options. One of the first considerations is often to decide on the location of treatment – that is, whether it can be carried out in the community or whether it is necessary to admit a patient to hospital. The decision to admit to hospital usually depends on the extent to which:

- The illness is interfering with a patient's functioning at home.
- Their health may deteriorate without rapid treatment or nursing care.
- They may pose a risk to themselves or to other people.

Treatment options are then considered in terms of physical treatments, psychological treatments and social treatments. In most cases, all three of these are important.

The final question asks about prognosis and the likely course of the disorder. Many psychiatric disorders have a wide range of prognoses. It is important to have a clear knowledge of those factors that may allow you to make judgements about prognosis in individual cases, so that you can educate and inform patients, and make appropriate decisions with regard to ongoing treatment.

The questions in the Clinical cases section of Chapter 4 are different. This chapter is specifically concerned with managing chronic disorders. Therefore, the diagnoses are given and the questions only ask about the three forms of treatment – physical, psychological and social.

The OSCE counselling questions ask how to approach other forms of common clinical situations, perhaps involving discussions with patients or their carers, or liaison with other medical specialties. These important aspects of clinical practice are increasingly being tested in clinical examinations.

Abbreviations

CBT	cognitive behavioural therapy
CPN	community psychiatric nurse
CT	computed tomography
ECG	electrocardiogram/electrocardiography
ECT	electroconvulsive therapy
EEG	electroencephalography
FBC	full blood count
GP	General Practitioner
i.m.	intramuscular
i.v.	intravenous
LFT	liver function test
MDMA	methylenedioxymethamphetamine or 'Ecstasy'
MHA	Mental Health Act 1983
MMSE	(Folstein's) Mini Mental State Examination
MRI	magnetic resonance imaging
MSE	mental state examination
OCD	obsessive–compulsive disorder
PTSD	post-traumatic stress disorder
SSRI	selective serotonin reuptake inhibitor
TCA	tricyclic antidepressant
TFT	thyroid function tests
U&Es	urea and electrolytes

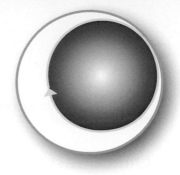

1 Psychosis

Clinical cases

For each of the case scenarios given, consider the following:

Q1: What is the likely differential diagnosis?
Q2: What information in the history supports the diagnosis, and what other information would help to confirm it?
Q3: What might the important aetiological factors be?
Q4: What treatment options are available?
Q5: What is the prognosis in this case?

CASE 1.1 – **Gradual onset of paranoid symptoms**

A 24-year-old biology graduate is referred to the outpatient department by his general practitioner (GP). He attends with his mother, who has been becoming increasingly concerned about him for some time. He tells you that he is feeling fine in himself. Objectively, you notice that he has reduced spontaneous movements, his tone of voice is monotonous and soft in volume. There is some suggestion that he is defensive or suspicious as he often asks you the reason for your questions and refuses to answer some personal questions. His mood is flat, showing little reactivity during the course of the interview, but he denies feeling depressed. He denies any psychotic symptoms and you are unable to detect any thought disorder.

His mother tells you that she began to worry 2 years ago after he finished his university degree course. He had previously been a high achiever, both academically and socially, with many friends and a hectic social life. However, since returning from university with a disappointing third class degree, he had made no efforts to gain any job and seemed to have lost contact with all of his friends. He was spending all of his time alone, often remaining upstairs in his bedroom for hours on end and interacting less and less with his family. More recently, he had begun to express some odd ideas, suggesting that someone was watching him and that other people knew where he was and what he was doing. His personal hygiene has begun to deteriorate, and he now refuses to allow his mother to clean his bedroom, which is becoming increasingly cluttered and dirty.

CASE 1.2 – **Acute-onset florid psychosis**

You are asked urgently to assess a 24-year-old woman who has recently moved to a large city to find work. She previously lived in a small rural community, and has had difficulty adapting to city life and finding employment. She gave up her job 2 weeks ago because it was not the sort of thing she was used to. Her boyfriend describes her as becoming 'increasingly anxious' throughout the last week, and her conversation increasingly confused and difficult to follow. She has not been sleeping well at night, often staying up doing housework all night and then sleeping during the day. For the 2 days prior to admission her behaviour had become extremely bizarre. She began to talk about people being hidden in the roof of her flat, saying that she could hear them sneezing and coughing, and could smell them as they passed in and out of the building. At one stage she said that she was a goddess who had been chosen to rid the world of evil. Sometimes she seemed happy, sometimes sad, and often very anxious and tense.

On the day before admission, she spent hours sitting almost motionless in a chair doing nothing, and then suddenly became agitated, running around and trying to do everything at once.

CASE 1.3 – **Low mood and symptoms of psychosis**

A 37-year-old woman is referred for an urgent assessment by her GP. She has been complaining of low mood for the past 3 months, and in recent weeks this has become increasingly severe. She has begun to complain that she can hear the voices of dead relatives talking to her, telling her that she would be better off dead, and that she is a useless wife and mother. She complains of a constant unpleasant smell, which she believes comes from her. She refuses to leave the house because she thinks other people will smell it. She has told her husband that the world is coming to an end, and has suggested that she has in some way caused this. Her GP has prescribed an antidepressant, but with no effect.

CASE 1.4 – **Long history of persecutory ideas**

A 45-year-old man is referred to the outpatient department by his GP. The man says that over recent months he has become increasingly low in mood. He says that he is under intolerable pressure because of persecution by his neighbours. It transpires that for over 20 years he has had to move house very frequently because someone keeps telling his neighbours that he is a paedophile. He denies this, and has no such convictions. He says that as a result, all of his neighbours are against him and spy on him to try to 'catch him at it' and drive him away. He thought that he had escaped when he moved into his current address 18 months ago, but now his persecutor has caught up with him again. He says that he cannot face moving away again.

His GP has confirmed that he has changed address many times over the last decade or so, but has otherwise lead a relatively normal life. He presents as a 'prickly' man, with few friends or social networks.

CASE 1.5 – **Unusual thoughts and behaviour associated with stimulant misuse**

Two friends bring a previously healthy 21-year-old man to the GP's surgery. He had been behaving in an increasingly odd way over the previous three days, becoming suspicious and irritable. He had started a university course 2 years previously, and had always been 'the life and soul of the party', going to nightclubs several nights each week. More recently, he had appeared angry and told his friends that he was being persecuted. When he was interviewed he was restless and frightened, and said that he had heard voices commenting on his actions and abusing him. He had heard references to himself on the radio and on television, and was concerned that people were following him.

CASE 1.6 – **Long-standing eccentric or unusual behaviour**

A GP asks you to visit a patient at home following concern from his family, after the death of his mother. He has always been a loner, preferring to be by himself than with others. When his sister told him that his mother had died, he showed little emotion, and attended her funeral in jeans and a dirty T-shirt, much to the family's disgust. He had always been quiet and compliant as a child, and seemed neither to seek nor to enjoy the company of other children. He currently lives alone and spends all of his time repairing electrical appliances.

ᴀ̇ᴀ̇ OSCE counselling cases

OSCE COUNSELLING CASE 1.1

You have seen a man suffering from a relapse of schizophrenia. He does not think that he requires treatment.

Q1: What factors would you take into account in deciding whether or not to use the Mental Health Act 1983?

Q2: What section of the Act would you use?

OSCE COUNSELLING CASE 1.2

You are asked to see a woman who gave birth to her first child 7 days previously. Her husband has told you that initially everything seemed fine, but that she began sleeping poorly on day 3. Over the past 4 days her mood has become increasingly labile, crying one minute, elated the next. She seems confused and he cannot hold a proper conversation with her as 'she just doesn't seem all there'. Her behaviour is grossly erratic and at times she seems to be seeing things or hearing things that are not present. You decide that the most likely diagnosis is puerperal psychosis.

Q1: What issues would you want to explore?

Q2: What would you tell the husband about his wife's condition?

Key concepts

In order to work through the core clinical cases in this chapter, you will need to understand the following key concepts.

The syndrome of psychosis is recognized by the presence of particular symptoms:

- Delusions: a belief which is held unshakeably despite evidence to the contrary, and which is not culturally appropriate. It is usually false, and is often considered to be of great personal significance by the patient.
- Hallucinations: a perception which arises in the absence of any external stimulus. It may occur in any sensory modality, though auditory are most common in psychiatric disorders.
- Passivity phenomena: the patient feels as though he or she is controlled externally by some other agency (i.e. they are passive). This may affect their thought processes (e.g. thought insertion, thought withdrawal, made feelings, made impulses) or their body (e.g. made actions, delusion of passivity associated with a somatic hallucination).

In general, these symptoms are always pathological. The only exceptions to this are some types of hallucination occurring in special situations, such as those associated with sleep (hypnagogic and hypnopompic). In these non-pathological situations, it is usual for the individual to retain insight and to recognize that these are not true or real experiences. In psychosis, this is not usually the case.

Symptoms of psychosis may occur in the context of an enormous range of illnesses, both psychiatric and physical. There are four non-affective psychoses, or primary psychotic illnesses, which are defined and recognized by the associated psychosis itself (see Table 1.1).

Table 1.1 Non-affective psychoses, or primary psychotic illnesses

Condition	Characteristics
Schizophrenia	A chronic illness characterized by repeated episodes of psychosis, particularly Schneider's first rank symptoms
	In addition, patients may experience negative symptoms, which are not episodic. Once present, they usually remain and gradually worsen
Schizoaffective disorder	The simultaneous presence of both typical symptoms of schizophrenia and affective disorder, neither being predominant
Persistent delusional disorder	At least 3 months' duration of one or more delusions. Other psychotic symptoms and negative symptoms of schizophrenia are absent
Acute and transient psychosis	Sudden onset of rapidly changing symptoms of florid psychosis. A strong mood element is common. The episode is often apparently precipitated by some stressful event. Usually lasts for no longer than 3 months, and often much less

The diagnosis may change over time. For example, an individual may present with a clinical picture suggestive of acute and transient psychosis. The psychosis may then persist for more than 3 months, and more typical symptoms of schizophrenia may develop. The diagnosis, prognosis and management may then be changed accordingly.

As with other psychiatric syndromes, the treatment of psychosis must take account of pharmacological, psychological and social interventions. However, the mainstay of treatment is usually pharmacological.

SCHNEIDER'S FIRST RANK SYMPTOMS OF SCHIZOPHRENIA

These are symptoms of psychosis which, if present, are considered to be suggestive of schizophrenia (see Table 1.2). However, they may occur in other types of psychosis and some patients with schizophrenia do not experience them.

Table 1.2 Schneider's first rank symptoms of schizophrenia

Type of auditory hallucination	Passivity of thought	Other passivity phenomena	One type of delusion
Thought echo perception	Thought broadcast	Made actions	Delusional
Running commentary	Thought insertion	Made feelings or sensations	
Discussing the patient	Thought withdrawal	Made impulses	

NEGATIVE SYMPTOMS OF SCHIZOPHRENIA

These symptoms tend to develop gradually and progressively, in contrast to the episodic nature of acute psychosis. They may severely impair an individual's ability to function in interpersonal relationships, work and leisure, and also limit independence.

These symptoms include:

- Impaired motivation.
- Lack of drive and initiative.
- Social withdrawal and loss of interest in other people.
- Emotional bluntness and reduced reactivity.
- Poverty of speech.
- Self-neglect.

OTHER PSYCHIATRIC CAUSES OF PSYCHOSIS

Psychosis may complicate affective disorder, whether depressive or manic, and usually indicates that the illness is severe. Patients with personality disorder are more likely to experience psychotic mental illness than other people.

Drug or alcohol misuse may lead to psychotic symptoms, and substance misuse is commonly co-morbid with psychotic mental illness. There are two reasons for this:

- Intoxication with some drugs causes psychosis; this is particularly likely with amphetamines and other stimulants. In these cases, the psychosis will resolve once the drug has been cleared from the body, and no specific psychiatric treatment is required.
- Drug misuse may precipitate an episode of psychosis in patients who have a mental illness such as schizophrenia. In these cases, the psychosis may persist after the patient has stopped using the drug.

It is often very difficult to distinguish between these two situations when someone presents with a psychosis. Short periods of assessment without any psychiatric medication or illegal substances may help to clarify. 'Drug-induced psychosis' is a commonly used term, but it is unclear which of the two situations it refers to. Therefore, it is best avoided.

PHYSICAL CAUSES OF PSYCHOSIS

Medical conditions which may cause psychosis include:

- Any cause of delirium.
- Head injury, or other intracranial pathology.
- Degenerating dementias.
- Epilepsy.
- Acute intermittent porphyria.
- Hyperthyroidism.

Answers

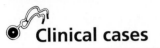
Clinical cases

CASE 1.1 – Gradual onset of paranoid symptoms

A1: What is the likely differential diagnosis?

Preferred diagnosis:

- Schizophrenia.

Alternative diagnoses:

- Drug misuse.
- Affective disorder.
- Personality disorder.
- No mental disorder.
- Organic causes of psychosis.

A2: What information in the history supports the diagnosis, and what other information would help to confirm it?

- This classical history of personal and social deterioration, together with the gradual development of persecutory ideas, is strongly suggestive of schizophrenia. Schizophrenia would be further suggested by the presence of first rank symptoms and a family history of schizophrenia.
- A similar deterioration in personal and social functioning may accompany habitual substance misuse. A drug history will help to exclude substance misuse as the primary cause, though you may wish to take a urine sample for urinalysis.
- The patient's flat mood and lack of interest/energy could be consistent with depression, though the very gradual and insidious decline is not typical. An affective disorder would be suggested by the presence of sustained and pervasive abnormality of mood and biological symptoms of depression or thought disorder characteristic of mania.
- Personality disorder is unlikely because of the clear change in his condition. A personality disorder would not have been preceded by a period of normal functioning in adolescence.
- It is possible that after attending university he has returned home with different values and opinions from those of his parents. They may be over-concerned and trying to find a medical explanation for their deteriorating relationship with their son. The severity of his problems makes this unlikely.
- Finally, in any new presentation it is important to consider physical diagnoses. It is unlikely that any endocrine, metabolic or intracranial neoplastic pathology would cause such a characteristic presentation. A reasonable screen for physical disorder, which will also provide a baseline for future antipsychotic treatment would be:
  - a physical examination;
  - full blood count (FBC), urea and electrolytes (U&Es), liver function tests (LFTs) and thyroid function tests (TFTs).
- Magnetic resonance imaging (MRI) of the head should be considered in all first presentations of psychosis to rule out an underlying physical disorder.
- An electroencephalogram (EEG) is unnecessary unless epilepsy or delirium is suspected.

A3: What might the important aetiological factors be?

PREDISPOSING FACTORS

Ask about history of birth trauma, delayed developmental milestones, positive family history.

PRECIPITATING FACTORS

This is difficult because of the insidious onset, but people with psychosis report more life events in the previous 3 months than those without psychosis. Leaving university and returning to his parents' home may be important.

MAINTAINING FACTORS

Drug misuse is common. Ongoing problems or stresses, such as pressure from well-meaning parents may also be important.

A4: What treatment options are available?

LOCATION

- Advantages of inpatient treatment:
  - reduction of risk of harm to self or to others;
  - improved observation and monitoring of symptoms;
  - more intensive development of therapeutic relationship and education about illness and need for treatment;
  - gives his family a rest, or removes him from the influence of a difficult family environment.
- If inpatient treatment is necessary, and the patient declines, the Mental Health Act (MHA) could be used. Admission under the MHA can also be considered if he refuses to accept medication. This has the potential disadvantage of jeopardizing your therapeutic relationship.
- In practice, you may be prepared to forego treatment for a short period, during which you would attempt to explain his illness and the importance of treatment. However, this period should be short because duration of untreated psychosis is important in determining future prognosis.
- If you treat him as an outpatient, he will need frequent outpatient medical review and a community psychiatric nurse (CPN) who can monitor his response and begin to develop a therapeutic relationship.

PHYSICAL

- Once you are satisfied that he is developing a psychosis, it is important to start treatment with an antipsychotic as soon as possible.
- Delay in treatment is associated with a worse prognosis.

PSYCHOLOGICAL

Initially, psychological treatment is likely to be supportive, attempting to develop a therapeutic relationship, educating him about his illness, and helping him to understand the importance of antipsychotic treatment.

SOCIAL

A social worker may be able to offer help and advice with respect to finances, appropriate occupation or employment. Attendance at a day hospital may facilitate these aspects of the patient's care.

A5: What is the prognosis in this case?

- The prognosis of schizophrenia is extremely variable, reflecting the heterogeneous nature of the disorder.

- In general, psychosis responds well to antipsychotic treatment, and the patient's condition should improve.
- However, schizophrenia is a lifelong condition, in which negative symptoms tend to develop gradually, and episodes of psychosis occur repeatedly.
- Suicide occurs in 10 per cent of cases, and is more likely in young men of previous high functioning, early in the course of the disorder.
- Good prognostic indicators include:
  - good family support;
  - normal premorbid personality;
  - high premorbid intelligence;
  - negative family history.
- Poor prognostic indicators include:
  - insidious onset with no precipitating factor;
  - male gender;
  - long duration of illness prior to treatment;
  - substance misuse;
  - lack of social support;
  - family history of schizophrenia;
  - young age of onset.

CASE 1.2 – **Acute-onset florid psychosis**

A1: What is the likely differential diagnosis?

Preferred diagnosis:

- Acute and transient psychotic disorder.

Alternative diagnoses:

- Drug intoxication.
- Manic episode.
- Schizophrenia.
- Physical causes of psychosis.

A2: What information in the history supports the diagnosis, and what other information would help to confirm it?

- The history is of a psychotic episode of acute (less than 2 weeks) onset. This appears to be characterized by florid, rapidly changing (polymorphic) symptoms and a marked affective component (though without the persistent change in mood typical of an affective psychosis) which did not precede the psychosis. There is some suggestion that it is associated with significant stresses relating to the patient's move away from home and difficulty finding appropriate employment. These features are typical of acute psychotic disorders.
- Acute florid psychoses may occur as a result of intoxication with drugs of abuse. Amphetamines are particularly likely to cause this. It is difficult to make this diagnosis on clinical grounds unless you are aware that the person has been misusing drugs. Visual perceptual abnormalities suggest psychosis due to drug intoxication. Ask carefully about drug use, and take a sample of urine for analysis.
- The diagnosis could be a manic episode, but a more prolonged period of deteriorating mood prior to the onset of psychosis would be usual. Ask carefully about this and any family history of mood disorders or other psychiatric disorders.
- Schizophrenia is unlikely because there are no first rank symptoms of schizophrenia described, the mood element seems too marked, and the duration of psychosis is not currently long enough. You would need to enquire about prodromal symptoms. It is possible that the episode is more longstanding than seems immediately apparent.

- Physical illnesses should always be considered, particularly epilepsy, head injury/intracranial tumours and encephalitis, endocrine and metabolic systemic illness. Psychosis may also be caused by certain medications such as L-dopa, steroid hormones, disulfiram and some anticonvulsants. You need to ask about the woman's past medical history, and any current treatment.

A3: What might the important aetiological factors be?

PREDISPOSING FACTORS

There may be evidence of an abnormal premorbid personality, particularly previous problems coping with stresses or difficulties in life. Check for a family history of psychiatric disorder.

PRECIPITATING FACTORS

These disorders are conceptualized as being precipitated by stressful events. This patient has been struggling to cope with a new lifestyle in a new environment, perhaps with little social network or support.

MAINTAINING FACTORS

The precipitating factors are ongoing and therefore are also maintaining factors. Substance misuse may also maintain symptoms.

A4: What treatment options are available?

LOCATION

- The vignette describes an acute, severe and unpredictable illness. Such a patient must be treated in hospital.
- If she does not consent to inpatient treatment, then an assessment for detention under the MHA should be considered. This is because:
  - there is a risk of self-harm because of her psychosis and associated chaotic behaviour;
  - there may be a risk of harm to others if she tries to defend herself against her persecutors;
  - her health is likely to deteriorate further without treatment.

PHYSICAL

- Antipsychotic medication will treat her psychosis over a period of weeks.
- In the meantime, symptomatic treatments may be necessary:
  - benzodiazepines may reduce anxiety levels and help to control very disturbed behaviour;
  - sedative antipsychotics may treat the psychosis as well as reduce anxiety;
  - hypnotics may help her to sleep at night.
- After recovery, she will need continuation antipsychotic treatment for at least 1 year to prevent relapse.
- Further maintenance treatment can be discussed with the patient. In general terms, the more her illness resembles schizophrenia, the greater the chances of recurrence and the more beneficial maintenance treatment will be. If the initial episode was typically schizophrenic, you may wish to recommend antipsychotic maintenance for up to 3 years.

PSYCHOLOGICAL

- Reassurance, explanation of symptoms and the development of a therapeutic relationship to promote compliance with treatment.
- After recovery, assessment of her personality may reveal personality traits that contributed to the onset of psychosis. It may be possible to work with her to improve her resilience to stress by improving low self-esteem, developing interpersonal skills, problem solving or anxiety management.

SOCIAL

This aims to re-establish her in the community while reducing some of the pressures that she has experienced previously.

A5: What is the prognosis in this case?

- The short-term prognosis of these disorders is good, the psychosis usually not lasting for more than 2/3 months and often much less.
- Patients will be at an increased risk of experiencing further episodes when compared with the general population. These episodes will be more likely to occur at times of stress.
- Recurrence is less likely if maintenance antipsychotic treatment is continued.

CASE 1.3 – **Low mood and symptoms of psychosis**

A1: What is the likely differential diagnosis?

Preferred diagnosis:

- Severe depressive episode with psychotic symptoms. This may:
  - be a first episode;
  - follow previous depressive episodes only (recurrent depressive disorder);
  - follow previous manic episodes (bipolar affective disorder).

Alternative diagnoses:

- Schizophrenia.
- Physical causes of psychosis.

A2: What information in the history supports the diagnosis, and what other information would help to confirm it?

- There seems to be a clear period of low mood preceding the onset of psychosis, the symptoms of which are typically depressive in origin (negative/insulting auditory hallucinations, unpleasant olfactory hallucinations and pessimistic ideas/delusions about the world accompanied by a sense of guilt). A full history and mental state examination (MSE) should uncover a depressive syndrome, probably with biological symptoms, and there may be a personal or family history of affective disorder.
- Check for first rank symptoms of schizophrenia, though if the depressive syndrome is present, the appropriate diagnosis will remain depression.
- Physical causes of psychosis should also be considered. Thyroid disease may cause mood disorder and, occasionally, psychosis. Olfactory hallucinations may be associated with seizures with a temporal lobe focus, but you would expect the symptoms to be clearly episodic. In addition, check current medications and basic physical investigations.

A3: What might the important aetiological factors be?

PREDISPOSING FACTORS

A personal or family history of mood disorder.

PRECIPITATING FACTORS

Life events or stressors, physical illness, particularly some systemic infections.

MAINTAINING FACTORS

Ongoing stressors or illness, poor compliance with antidepressant medication.

A4: What treatment options are available?

LOCATION

- Admission to hospital is necessary because she is severely depressed and therefore vulnerable to self-neglect and self-harm.
- An attempt should be made to persuade her to accept admission voluntarily, but if this is impossible the MHA should be considered.

PHYSICAL

- Depressive episodes with psychotic symptoms require combination treatment with an antidepressant and an antipsychotic. Neither treatment alone is as effective. This combination should be effective over a period of weeks.
- If a very rapid response is required (for example she is not eating or drinking or is actively attempting to harm herself), electroconvulsive therapy (ECT) should be considered. ECT is more effective in patients with depression who also have psychotic symptoms or biological symptoms of depression.
- After recovery from the acute episode the antipsychotic medication may be gradually withdrawn. Continuation and maintenance antidepressant treatment must be considered and discussed with the patient. If this is her first episode, the antidepressant should be continued for at least 6 months, and given the severity of the episode it may be continued for longer.
- If she has had previous episodes she needs long-term maintenance antidepressant treatment.

PSYCHOLOGICAL

- Support, reassurance and explanation of symptoms.
- Cognitive therapy, while effective in mild to moderate depression, is less effective in severe depression. There may be a role for this as she recovers.
- After recovery, personality assessment may indicate areas that can be worked on psychologically. Problem-solving therapy, assertiveness training, anxiety management or cognitive or dynamic psychotherapy may be useful to improve her resilience and ability to cope with stress. This in turn may reduce the risk of depressive episodes being precipitated by stressful events in the future.

SOCIAL

Social support may be useful in some patients to ease their return to the community while they may still be vulnerable to relapse.

A5: What is the prognosis in this case?

- The short-term prognosis of depressive episodes is good. Response to treatment is usual.
- However, depression is a relapsing illness and she is likely to have further episodes in the future.
- The likelihood of recurrence is reduced by maintenance antidepressant treatment.

CASE 1.4 – **Long history of persecutory ideas**

A1: What is the likely differential diagnosis?

Preferred diagnosis:

- Persistent delusional disorder.

Alternative diagnoses:

- Personality disorder – probably paranoid.
- Schizophrenia.
- Depressive episode.
- Physical causes of psychosis.

A2: What information in the history supports the diagnosis, and what other information would help to confirm it?

- The long-standing nature of his systematized abnormal beliefs suggests a persistent delusional disorder. To confirm the diagnosis, you must establish that the beliefs are delusional and have been present for over 3 months.
- Such long-standing difficulties may also represent a personality disorder – probably a paranoid personality disorder. If the beliefs are overvalued ideas, personality disorder is likely. However, if the beliefs are delusions, personality disorder cannot be the sole diagnosis, though it is often comorbid with a delusional disorder.
- Schizophrenia may be excluded by demonstrating the absence of first rank symptoms.
- Depression may be excluded as a primary diagnosis by demonstrating the absence of a depressive syndrome, or by demonstrating that the psychosis developed before the mood disorder.
- Physical causes are very unlikely in such a long-standing disorder.

A3: What might the important aetiological factors be?

PREDISPOSING FACTORS

Persistent delusional disorder commonly occurs in people with an abnormal personality – usually a paranoid personality disorder.

PRECIPITATING FACTORS

It will be difficult to identify precipitating factors, as the symptoms have been present for so long.

MAINTAINING FACTORS

Maintaining factors related to his personality and lifestyle may be difficult to modify. For example, his persecutory beliefs are likely to increase his isolation from other people which will in turn fuel his beliefs.

A4: What treatment options are available?

LOCATION

- Because of his low mood and persecutory beliefs, you must consider his risk of self-harm and the risk of harm to others. If these are assessed as high, then inpatient treatment may be necessary.
- He may want to spend a period away from home, to give himself a break from his persecution, though his delusional beliefs may transfer themselves to nurses or other patients in hospital.
- In practice, outpatient treatment should be possible with close monitoring by a CPN.

PHYSICAL

- He has a psychosis – therefore, a trial of treatment with an antipsychotic is necessary.
- If he has a comorbid depressive illness, an antidepressant may be useful in combination.

PSYCHOLOGICAL

- Discouragement of maladaptive coping strategies, such as alcohol misuse or not going out of the house, is an important first step, together with an attempt to establish a trusting relationship.
- Cognitive therapy may then modify his abnormal beliefs. The aim is probably not to 'cure' him of his beliefs, but to attempt to reduce their intensity and the impact that they have on his life and functioning.

SOCIAL

To improve his social networks and reduce his isolation.

A5: What is the prognosis in this case?

- The prognosis of persistent delusional disorder is poor. The psychosis is likely to remain present indefinitely, despite treatment. Treatment may be successful in reducing his preoccupation with his symptoms.
- Many patients who present with persistent delusional disorder subsequently develop schizophrenia.
- Poor prognostic factors include:
  - the length of time the delusions have been present;
  - abnormal previous personality;
  - poor social networks.
- Good prognostic factors include presence of symptoms of depression, as this can be readily treated.

CASE 1.5 – Unusual thoughts and behaviour associated with stimulant misuse

A1: What is the likely differential diagnosis?

Preferred diagnosis:

- Intoxication with stimulant drugs.

Alternative diagnoses:

- Schizophrenia.
- Delirium due to drug withdrawal.
- Mania.

A2: What information in the history supports the diagnosis, and what other information would help to confirm it?

The club scene is strongly associated with the use of stimulant and hallucinogenic drugs such as amphetamines and Ecstasy (MDMA). Intoxication with these may cause acute psychosis. If the symptoms are caused by intoxication, they will gradually fade over the next 2–7 days as the effects of the drugs wear off. A careful MSE should be repeated every day or so to monitor progress. A urinary drug screen would be useful to determine what he has taken, but amphetamines, cocaine or MDMA will only be detectable in the urine for 2–3 days after the last dose.

- The key task is to distinguish an episode of psychosis caused by intoxication from an episode of severe mental illness precipitated by the drugs. The mention of voices commenting on his actions should be carefully explored as this may be a first rank symptom of schizophrenia, and may be an early sign of the development of the disorder. A positive family history or a more prolonged onset over a period of weeks may suggest schizophrenia. Independent information must be sought.
- Mania may present with restlessness and persecutory beliefs. A family history of affective disorder and a clear episode of increasingly elated mood prior to the onset of psychosis would support this.
- A detailed drug history should be obtained, including details of amounts used and duration of use, route of use, and evidence of dependence.

A3: What might the important aetiological factors be?

PREDISPOSING FACTORS

A family history of psychosis may indicate that he has a low threshold for developing such symptoms.

PRECIPITATING FACTORS

The disorder has been precipitated by stimulant intoxication. The history may show you that for some reason he has been using more than usual in recent days or weeks.

MAINTAINING FACTORS

If the psychosis is simply due to stimulant intoxication then it will not continue once the stimulants have been cleared from the body.

A4: What treatment options are available?

LOCATION

- Dependent on assessment of risk factors such as:
  - the severity of symptoms;
  - likely diagnosis;
  - available support;
  - violence or self-harm;
  - past history of similar episodes;
  - attitude to symptoms and treatment.
- He is presenting with psychotic symptoms and appears in a vulnerable state, and ideally would not be left alone. Therefore, admission to psychiatric hospital is likely. This will allow better support and observation.
- If he refuses admission and there is a risk of harm to self or others, use of the MHA may be considered.
- It may be possible to manage him at home if he has good support from family or friends who will stay with him 24 h a day.

PHYSICAL

- If the symptoms are purely due to intoxication they will fade over the next 48 h, without medication.
- However, a small dose of benzodiazepines may be helpful to aid sleep and to reduce agitation.
- If the psychosis persists, suggesting a severe mental illness, antipsychotic medication should be started.

PSYCHOLOGICAL

A clear explanation of the likely cause of the symptoms is necessary, combined with reassurance and support during the first 24–48 h.

SOCIAL

Social support by way of employment training, financial help and accommodation may help to avoid substance misuse in the future.

A5: What is the prognosis in this case?

If the symptoms are caused by intoxication, the psychotic symptoms will resolve within 2–7 days.

CASE 1.6 – Long-standing eccentric or unusual behaviour

A1: What is the likely differential diagnosis?

Preferred diagnosis:

- Personality disorder – probably schizoid.

Alternative diagnoses:

- Schizophrenia.
- Depressive disorder.
- Social phobia.
- Asperger's syndrome.

A2: What information in the history supports the diagnosis, and what other information would help to confirm it?

- The history suggests that many of his problems have been present persistently since his childhood. This may suggest a personality disorder. To confirm this you need to demonstrate that the presentation:
  - has been present continuously since adolescence;
  - is inflexible, occurring in a wide range of situations;
  - is an extreme deviation from normal in that culture;
  - is associated with personal distress or problems in social functioning.
- The preference for solitary activities, emotional coldness, insensitivity to social norms or conventions and eccentric solitary hobbies suggests schizoid personality disorder. Other features to look for would include indifference to praise or criticism from others and a preoccupation with fantasy or introspection. In particular, you would want to demonstrate that he has no desire for interpersonal relationships (rather than wanting them but being unable to form them).
- The early stages (or prodrome) of schizophrenia may be similar. However, you would expect a period of more normal functioning at some time in the past. You must ensure there are no psychotic symptoms, which would exclude personality disorder as the diagnosis.
- In depression a more acute onset and previous normal functioning would be expected. You should specifically exclude a depressive syndrome, as people with personality disorder are more likely to have such disorders.
- Asperger's syndrome would be suggested by a history of problems with social interaction and restricted repetitive patterns of interests and behaviours since early childhood.

A3: What might the important aetiological factors be?

PREDISPOSING FACTORS

Personality disorders are multifactorial in aetiology, with both genetic and environmental influences being of relevance. There may have been some relative who was similarly eccentric.

PRECIPITATING FACTORS

His presentation has been precipitated by the death of his mother, under which circumstances his personality disorder appears even more inappropriate than at other times.

MAINTAINING FACTORS

Personality disorders are intrinsically enduring.

A4: What treatment options are available?

LOCATION

- Patients with personality disorder rarely do well when admitted to hospital, where their idiosyncratic lifestyle may fit in poorly.
- Therefore, any treatment will be as an outpatient unless he also has a comorbid mental illness.

PHYSICAL

There is no role for drugs in the treatment of schizoid personality disorder.

PSYCHOLOGICAL

- Attempts to treat personality disorder depend on the establishment of a good therapeutic relationship. People with schizoid personality disorder have no desire or ability to form such relationships, usually do not complain of problems themselves, and rarely seek treatment. Therefore, these personality disorders are rarely treatable.

- Psychological treatment would aim to:
  - develop a therapeutic relationship;
  - encourage gradually increasing amounts of socialization;
  - support the family or carers;
  - improve self-esteem;
  - build on the individual's strengths;
  - discourage adverse activities such as substance misuse.

SOCIAL

Social support by way of employment training, financial help or help with accommodation may be useful in individual cases, depending on the wishes of the patient.

A5: What is the prognosis in this case?

- Personality disorders are chronic by definition, and schizoid personality disorder is particularly persistent.
- Improvement is unlikely unless his presentation has been contributed to by a comorbid mental illness such as depression.

🏃 OSCE counselling cases

OSCE COUNSELLING CASE 1.1

You have seen a man suffering from a relapse of schizophrenia. He does not think that he requires treatment.

A1: What factors would you take into account in deciding whether or not to use the Mental Health Act 1983?

You should consider the following issues:

- His history of compliance with outpatient care. If he has a long history of failing to comply with outpatient treatment when unwell he may be unlikely to comply now. This increases the likelihood of a deterioration in his health.
- The availability of community support. His carers at home should be consulted. Are they happy to continue to look after him, or are they struggling to cope under mounting pressure?
- Does his psychiatric history suggest that once medication is commenced his symptoms will respond quickly, or is it more likely that he will remain ill for some time, or even deteriorate further before eventually improving?
- If he remains as an outpatient, what measures are you able to put in place for treatment? (The crisis resolution home treatment team may be able to provide very frequent reviews, attendance at a day centre and other support.) Is he likely to comply with them? Are they likely to be sufficient?
- Does he currently have any thoughts of self-harm, depressive symptoms, ideas of hopelessness or psychotic symptoms suggesting that he may pose a risk to himself. Does he have any history of self-harm?
- Do any of his symptoms suggest that he may pose a risk of violence to others? If so, who? Does he have any history of being aggressive or violent when unwell or otherwise? Is he misusing drugs?

The basic legal requirements that make an individual liable to be detained are that:

- The person has a mental disorder of a nature or degree which makes it appropriate for him to be detained in hospital for medical treatment. Therefore, you need to consider the severity of illness:
  - What is the frequency and intensity of symptoms?
  - How distressing are they?
  - How preoccupied is he with them?
  - Are they affecting or influencing his behaviour?
  - How much insight does he have?
  - Will he be compliant with treatment?
- It is necessary for him to be detained for treatment in the interests of his/her own health or safety or for the protection of others.
  - Will admission prevent deterioration in his health?
  - Will admission prevent him from coming to harm through self-neglect or exploitation by others?
  - Will admission reduce the risk of self-harm or suicide?
  - Will admission reduce the risk of harm he poses to other people?
- There is appropriate medical treatment available: medical treatment in this case includes antipsychotic treatment but will also encompass nursing care, observations, restrictions to ensure safety of patient/others, and all other aspects of care and treatment for mental disorder.

A2: What section of the Act would you use?

In this situation, the most commonly used sections of the MHA1983 are Section 2 and Section 3:

- Section 2 is an assessment and treatment order lasting for a maximum of 28 days. It cannot be renewed, but can be converted to a section 3 treatment order if necessary.
- Section 3 is a treatment order lasting for an initial maximum of 6 months, which can be renewed for further periods of detention.
- You are likely to use Section 2 if:
  - the diagnosis is unclear;
  - there is no treatment plan in place and further assessment is required;
  - the patient is well known to you but his current presentation is atypical;
  - the patient has not previously been admitted to hospital or has not been in regular contact with psychiatric services.
- You are likely to use Section 3 if:
  - The patient has an established diagnosis and his current presentation is typical of his relapses.
  - There is a treatment plan in place based on previous episodes of illness.

OSCE COUNSELLING CASE 1.2

You are asked to see a woman who gave birth to her first child 7 days previously. Her husband has told you that initially everything seemed fine, but that she began sleeping poorly on day 3. Over the past 4 days her mood has become increasingly labile, crying one minute, elated the next. She seems confused and he cannot hold a proper conversation with her as 'she just doesn't seem all there'. Her behaviour is grossly erratic and at times she seems to be seeing things or hearing things that are not present. You decide that the most likely diagnosis is puerperal psychosis.

A1: What issues would you want to explore?

Consider the following issues.

- About the pregnancy:
  - Was it planned and wanted?
  - Were there any stresses or problems during it?
  - Was she ill or did it go smoothly?
  - Did she bond with the baby prenatally (stroke her tummy, talk to it, etc.)?
- About the birth:
  - Was this traumatic?
  - What was the level of medical intervention?
  - How did it compare to her expectations?
- About her relationship with her husband:
  - Does it seem mutually supportive?
  - Is he critical or controlling?
- About any previous personal or family history of psychiatric disorder.
- About her relationship with the baby:
  - Does she feel love for it?
  - Does she have any odd thoughts or delusions relating to the baby, or any ideas of harming it?
  - Does she play and talk to it?
  - Is she able to care for it?

A2: What would you tell the husband about his wife's condition?

Explain to the husband that:

- His wife is suffering from an acute serious mental illness.
- That this is not uncommon following childbirth, and that a full recovery can be confidently expected, but that she may become worse before she improves.
- Discuss the risks to the woman and the baby, and consider the location of treatment.

- The woman will almost certainly need to be admitted to a mother and baby unit as she should not be left alone at all at present. If necessary, the MHA can be used.
- There are two forms of treatment. Antipsychotic medication may be effective, but often these illnesses respond particularly well to ECT. Explain the nature of these treatments, with particular reference to breast-feeding.

REVISION PANEL

- The syndrome of psychosis may result from a wide range of physical and mental disorders.
- Psychiatric causes of psychosis may be separated into affective psychoses and non-affective psychoses. Establishing the presence or absence of an underlying pathological mood state is crucial to diagnosis.
- Psychosis may be associated with risk behaviours, to self and occasionally to others. Assessment of such risks is essential in all cases.
- Admission to hospital is necessary to treat severe or acute psychosis. The response to antipsychotic medication is likely to take some weeks.

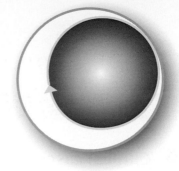

2 Mood disorders

Questions

Clinical cases

For each of the case scenarios given, consider the following:

> **Q1**: What is the likely differential diagnosis?
> **Q2**: What information in the history supports the diagnosis, and what other information would help to confirm it?
> **Q3**: What might the important aetiological factors be?
> **Q4**: What treatment options are available?
> **Q5**: What is the prognosis in this case?

CASE 2.1 – Low mood and anxiety without severe disturbance of functioning

A 40-year-old woman presents to her general practitioner (GP) complaining of feeling tired and 'washed-out'. She has had difficulty getting off to sleep for about 4 weeks, but has felt restless during the day. Straightforward, everyday tasks have become a challenge and sometimes provoke a dry mouth and churning stomach, but she occasionally feels tearful. The GP is aware that the woman's mother died 3 months prior to the presentation. The patient describes no thoughts of self-harm.

CASE 2.2 – Severe low mood impairing functioning

A 45-year-old man presents to his GP with feelings of hopelessness, sadness and helplessness. He says that he cries for no reason, and has difficulty sleeping. He noticed that the problems began about 6 weeks before, and he did not feel able to shrug them off. He has been drinking more alcohol than usual, and has stopped going to work. When on his own, he admitted that he had thought of driving his car into the local lake.

CASE 2.3 – Low mood after childbirth

A health visitor refers a 29-year-old teacher to the psychiatric team. The woman gave birth to her first baby just over a month ago, but has not felt well since. The pregnancy was unplanned, and the baby was premature, having to be nursed in the special care baby unit for 2 weeks. The teacher feels tearful all the time, tired and irritable. Her partner feels that she is not coping with looking after the baby, and the woman is scared that she has had fleeting thoughts of harming the infant.

CASE 2.4 – Overactivity, elation and grandiose ideas

A 27-year-old woman is brought to the local accident and emergency department by her family. She appears restless, pacing around the waiting room, and her parents say that she has recently been asked to leave her job. She has not slept for several nights, and her speech is rapid and quickly wanders off the point. She had recently purchased an expensive car, and makes references to being offered a new job as chief executive of a major company. She is very reluctant to remain in the A&E department because she has far too much to do and considers it a waste of everyone's time. She believes that she is far too important to be messed around in such a way.

☖ OSCE counselling cases

OSCE COUNSELLING CASE 2.1

You are about to commence a patient on antidepressant treatment.

Q1: What would you tell him about the drug, its mechanism of action and side effects?

Q2: Are there other options available if he refuses?

Key concepts

Mood disorders are characterized by episodes of persistent and severe elevation or depression of mood. These episodes of illness may be precipitated by stressful life events in an individual who has an intrinsic predisposition to mood disorder (often manifested in family history).

A depressive episode is characterized by three fundamental symptoms:

- Low mood.
- Lack of energy (anergia).
- Lack of interest in or enjoyment of normal activities (anhedonia).

A manic episode is characterized by:

- Elevation of mood.
- Increased energy and overactivity.

Historically, the classification of depression has been problematic, giving rise to a variety of confusing terms. Classifications such as endogenous versus reactive depression tried to draw a distinction between different causes of a depressive syndrome, but are not particularly helpful. It is better to think of depression as being a biologically driven disorder that may be precipitated by environmental stressors, but which leads to a common set of symptoms. The treatment response is not dependent on the cause.

These disorders are usually recurrent. An individual who has had more than one mood episode is diagnosed with recurrent depressive disorder if they have only had depressive episodes. If they have had one or more previous manic episodes, they are diagnosed with bipolar affective disorder (see Table 2.1). This is so even without depressive episodes, because people who have had mania are liable to develop depression.

Table 2.1 Episodes of illness related to diagnosis

Episodes of illness	Diagnosis
One episode of depression	Depressive episode
Two or more episodes of depression with no episodes of hypomania or mania	Recurrent depressive disorder
One episode of hypomania or mania	Hypomania or mania
More than one episode of hypomania or mania	Bipolar affective disorder
One or more episodes of hypomania or mania + one or more episodes of depression	Bipolar affective disorder

It is important to note that depression is under-recognized, particularly in primary care. Sometimes, doctors may be reluctant to treat depression because of the risk of deliberate overdose. However, modern antidepressants are relatively safe in overdose, and under-treatment of depression makes a more important contribution to suicide than overdose of prescribed antidepressants.

Answers

Clinical cases

CASE 2.1 – **Low mood and anxiety without severe disturbance of functioning**

A1: What is the likely differential diagnosis?

Preferred diagnosis:

- Mild depressive episode.

Alternative diagnoses:

- Adjustment disorder/bereavement.
- Generalized anxiety disorder.
- Physical problem.
- Alcohol misuse or dependence.

A2: What information in the history supports the diagnosis, and what other information would help to confirm it?

- A recent onset of low mood, tiredness and poor sleep are very suggestive of a depressive episode. The history and mental state examination (MSE) should look for the other symptoms of a depressive syndrome. It is important to explore the onset and severity of the symptoms. This may focus on any possible stressors, past history of psychiatric disorder, or a family history of psychiatric disorder.
- It may be difficult to distinguish between bereavement and a depressive syndrome. If persistent and severe symptoms or functional impairment remain present more than 3 months after the death, it is likely that a depressive episode has been precipitated. Bereavement may, however, vary greatly between cultures.
- Anxiety symptoms are commonly present in depression. If a depressive syndrome is present, then the diagnosis of generalized anxiety disorder is excluded.
- Blood tests may provide a useful baseline and exclude physical causes for some of the symptoms, for example anaemia (full blood count [FBC]), diabetes (blood glucose) or hypothyroidism (thyroid function tests [TFTs]).
- The possibility of alcohol or substance misuse must be considered, and the CAGE questionnaire (see p. 125) may be a useful screening tool. Prescribed medication should also be reviewed.

A3: What might the important aetiological factors be?

PREDISPOSING FACTORS

She may have a family history of depression or mood disorder. Other factors that may be important include lack of emotional support or death of a parent in childhood, the lack of a supportive partner and having several young children at home.

PRECIPITATING FACTORS

It seems likely that the depressive episode has been precipitated by the death of her mother.

MAINTAINING FACTORS

Personality traits such as anxiety, obsessionality, ineffectual coping strategies for stress and low self-esteem may be important in maintaining her symptoms.

A4: What treatment options are available?

LOCATION

This problem is best treated in the community, probably in primary care.

PHYSICAL

- A short-term course of hypnotic medication for night sedation may be useful, but should not be provided without other interventions.
- There may be a role for antidepressant medication, which should continue for 6 months after full recovery.

PSYCHOLOGICAL

- Initial treatment may centre on reassurance and provision of information.
- Problem-solving strategies can be taught, and anxiety management skills developed.

SOCIAL

Tackling problems such as unsuitable housing, financial difficulties or child care may help to reduce stresses that could jeopardize response to treatment.

A5: What is the prognosis in this case?

- Mild depressive episodes usually respond well to simple treatment.
- The outcome is likely to depend on the severity of any life events that have preceded this episode, the patient's predominant personality traits, and the existence or otherwise of a supportive or confiding relationship.

CASE 2.2 – **Severe low mood impairing functioning**

A1: What is the likely differential diagnosis?

Preferred diagnosis:

- Severe depressive disorder.

Alternative diagnoses:

- Alcohol or substance misuse/dependence.
- Physical disorder:
  - infectious disease – influenza, human immunodeficiency virus (HIV);
  - endocrine disorder – thyroid disorder, Cushing's syndrome;
  - neoplastic – lung, testicular, cerebral;
  - prescribed medication, e.g. corticosteroids, β-blockers, interferon.

A2: What information in the history supports the diagnosis, and what other information would help to confirm it?

This man has the three core symptoms of a depressive disorder – low mood, anergia and anhedonia. The history will explore the other symptoms of the depressive syndrome.

- Biological symptoms of depression:
  - marked loss of appetite;
  - weight loss (5 per cent in last month);

- marked loss of libido;
- disturbed sleep – waking in the morning 2 hours before the usual time;
- a diurnal variation in mood with depression worse in the morning;
- psychomotor retardation or agitation.
- Cognitive symptoms of depression:
  - reduced attention and concentration;
  - reduced self-confidence and self-esteem;
  - ideas of guilt and unworthiness;
  - pessimistic views of the future;
  - ideas or acts of self-harm or suicide.
- An interview with the man's wife or other close friends or family would help confirm the story. A review of his past medical records may reveal previous similar episodes and point to effective treatment strategies.
- A drug and alcohol history (and perhaps blood tests or urinalysis) should exclude this as a primary diagnosis.
- A review of any medications that he is taking.
- A physical examination and routine blood tests (FBC, liver function tests [LFTs], urea and electrolytes [U&Es] and TFTs) should be conducted to exclude physical causes for the symptoms.

A3: What might the important aetiological factors be?

PREDISPOSING FACTORS

A family history of mood disorder and an abnormal premorbid personality may be important.

PRECIPITATING FACTORS

Depressive episodes are commonly precipitated by a life event or stressor or may occur following physical illness, such as influenza virus infection.

MAINTAINING FACTORS

Ongoing social stressors, high alcohol consumption or lack of a supportive relationship may prevent resolution.

A4: What treatment options are available?

LOCATION

- Provided that his wife is willing to support him, he would be best treated at home.
- If a careful exploration of the man's suicidal ideation led you to believe that he was at risk of self-harm, it may be necessary to admit him to hospital.

PHYSICAL

- Antidepressant medication is the first-choice treatment.
- Because the therapeutic effect takes about 2 weeks to develop, short-term symptomatic treatment with a benzodiazepine for anxiety or a hypnotic may be considered.

PSYCHOLOGICAL

- Educate the patient and their family about the nature of depression, its cause and likely time-course.
- Cognitive therapy targets the negative thoughts that occur in depression (for example ideas of guilt, worthlessness, pessimism).
- Cognitive behavioural techniques such as problem-solving techniques or activity scheduling may be considered.

SOCIAL

Advice about financial difficulties, support with time off from work and attempts to resolve housing difficulties may all facilitate resolution of the problem.

A5: What is the prognosis in this case?

- The short-term prognosis of depressive episodes is good. About 75 per cent of cases respond to simple antidepressant treatment.
- However, the majority of people who experience a depressive episode will go on to have another one at some point in their life.
- Up to 10–15 per cent of severely depressed patients complete suicide.

CASE 2.3 – **Low mood after childbirth**

A1: What is the likely differential diagnosis?

Preferred diagnosis:

- Postnatal depression.

Alternative diagnosis:

- Baby blues.

A2: What information in the history supports the diagnosis, and what other information would help to confirm it?

- Childbirth is one of the most potent precipitants of mental illness. Postnatal depression occurs in 10 per cent of new mothers within 4–6 weeks of delivery. The clinical features are similar to those of depression (see above), although the baby is usually a central preoccupation. In addition to thoughts of self-harm, thoughts of harming the baby must be explored.
- In addition to the usual issues, it is important to consider whether the mother has bonded with her child, whether she is able to cope with the demands of looking after it, and what degree of family support she has with this. A history from the father is essential in order to understand his concerns and evaluate the social context of the illness.
- Over 50 per cent of mothers experience transient low mood and tearfulness (known as 'baby blues') on the third or fourth day postnatally, but these symptoms usually resolve within a few days with no treatment.

A3: What might the important aetiological factors be?

PREDISPOSING FACTORS

- A family history of mood disorder is important, but social factors are particularly relevant in the aetiology of this disorder:
  - increased age;
  - problems in relationship with mother/father-in-law;
  - marital conflict;
  - unplanned pregnancy or unwanted baby;
  - physical problems in pregnancy and perinatal period;
  - abnormal premorbid personality.

PRECIPITATING FACTORS

These are defined by the main precipitating factor – childbirth.

MAINTAINING FACTORS

Common maintaining factors are poor bonding with the baby, lack of a supportive relationship with partner, and problems coping with a baby who is naturally irritable or an infrequent sleeper.

A4: What treatment options are available?

LOCATION

- Most cases are managed at home.
- The opinion of the father is important.
- In the event of admission a mother-and-baby unit should be sought. Factors suggesting that inpatient treatment is necessary include:
  - a risk of neglect of the baby;
  - risk of self-harm;
  - risk of harming the baby;
  - inability to cope with the baby;
  - lack of social support.

PHYSICAL

- Postnatal depression responds well to treatment with antidepressants.
- Most antidepressants are excreted in breast milk, but may be used with caution.
- Electroconvulsive therapy is also particularly effective in postnatal illnesses, and may provide quicker resolution in severe cases.

PSYCHOLOGICAL

- Explanation and reassurance to the mother and her family are essential.
- Group settings that provide support from other depressed mothers may be beneficial.

SOCIAL

She should be encouraged to foster links with as many sources of support as possible – local mothers' groups, family, GP, midwife, health visitor.

A5: What is the prognosis in this case?

- Postnatal depression has a very good prognosis, and full recovery is usual.
- A worse prognosis may be suggested by abnormal premorbid personality and poor social support or marital problems.
- There is an increased risk of further depressive episodes, both following future pregnancy and at other times.

CASE 2.4 – **Overactivity, elation and grandiose ideas**

A1: What is the likely differential diagnosis?

Preferred diagnosis:

- Manic episode or bipolar affective disorder.

Alternative diagnoses:

- Acute and transient psychotic disorder.
- Stimulant intoxication.
- Physical disorders.
- Medication such as steroids.

A2: What information in the history supports the diagnosis, and what other information would help to confirm it?

The key features of mania are elevation of mood and increased energy and activity levels. In addition, this case demonstrates other common features such as grandiose ideas, decreased need for sleep and reckless spending. Other symptoms to elicit in a history and MSE may include feelings of physical and mental efficiency, increased sociability and talkativeness, poor attention and concentration and distractibility.

- Relevant factors in a full history include an assessment of risk of harm to self or others, and a personal or family history of depression or mania. It is important to ask her about use of stimulant drugs or prescribed medication. Look for rapid and pressured speech, flight of ideas, tangentiality and racing thoughts.
- The difference between hypomania and mania is one of degree of severity of symptoms. In hypomania the person is able to continue with normal work or leisure activities, but with some disruption. The patient with mania is unable to do so, and may also experience psychotic symptoms. Her belief that she has been offered a new job may suggest that the diagnosis is one of mania.
- If she has had a previous episode of mood disorder then the diagnosis would be bipolar affective disorder.
- In an acute and transient psychotic disorder, psychosis would be more prominent and elation and grandiosity less persistent.
- Intoxication with stimulants should be excluded by the history and perhaps by a urine drug screen.
- A physical examination is necessary to exclude severe dehydration, evidence of head injury or other physical disorders. Relevant investigations would include an FBC and U&Es.
- Review all medication as some can precipitate mania, for example steroids and antidepressants.

A3: What might the important aetiological factors be?

PREDISPOSING FACTORS

Bipolar affective disorder is strongly genetically determined, and a family history is likely.

PRECIPITATING FACTORS

Life events or stressors, lack of sleep or substance misuse may precipitate manic episodes. Non-compliance with mood-stabilizing prophylaxis is a common precipitant of manic episodes in bipolar affective disorder.

MAINTAINING FACTORS

Continued substance misuse or non-compliance with medication is common.

A4: What treatment options are available?

LOCATION

- Admission to hospital is essential. Mania is associated with:
  - a risk of self-harm, often due to unrealistic beliefs in one's abilities;
  - a risk of self-neglect;
  - deterioration without treatment.
- People with mania usually lack insight, particularly in their first episode, often claiming that they have never been so well. The MHA should be used if necessary.

PHYSICAL

- There are two treatment approaches:
  - antipsychotic medication is effective in treating acute mania. Its sedative effects may be useful before the antimanic effect occurs. In severe cases it may be given by the intramuscular route;
  - lithium and valproate are both mood stabilizers which are effective in acute mania, though with a delayed action.
- Benzodiazepines may be useful to provide short-term sedation.
- ECT is also effective, but is reserved for use in medication-resistant cases.

PSYCHOLOGICAL

- Explanation and reassurance are important for the patient and their family.
- Patients and their families can be taught to recognize early symptoms of relapse and formulate a management plan to prevent deterioration.
- After recovery, cognitive behavioural strategies aimed at improving resilience to stress and improving understanding of the disorder may be important.

SOCIAL

When the manic episode has resolved, the patient may be left with debts or other social problems that were created during the illness. Help in resolving these issues can improve compliance with medication and engagement with treatment services.

A5: What is the prognosis in this case?

- Some 90 per cent of people that experience a manic episode will have future recurrences without treatment.
- Up to 15 per cent of patients with bipolar disorder ultimately commit suicide.

👥 OSCE counselling cases

OSCE COUNSELLING CASE 2.1

You are about to commence a patient on antidepressant treatment.

A1: What would you tell him about the drug, its mechanism of action and side effects?

- There is a variety of antidepressant medication. The two classes most commonly used are selective serotonin reuptake inhibitors (SSRIs) and tricyclic antidepressants (TCAs).
- No antidepressant has been conclusively demonstrated to work more quickly or more effectively than the others.
- The side effect profile of the drug may be the most useful way of selecting which one to use in a particular case.
- Due to the nature of a depressive disorder the patient may not believe that anything will help them, and be anxious that they will become dependent or 'addicted' to any medication prescribed. You should talk positively about the benefits and likely success of antidepressant medication, and correct any misunderstandings about dependence on the drug.
- It should be made clear that the beneficial effects of the drug are unlikely to appear for at least 2–3 weeks. It is important that the patient continues to take the drug, even if initially they do not feel that it is helping them. They will need to take the drug for at least 6 weeks before evaluating its efficacy.
- It is important to describe the common side effects, explaining that these will come on almost immediately and be worst in the first 3–7 days. Typical side effects include:
  - SSRIs:
    - gastrointestinal upset, including nausea and diarrhoea;
    - headache;
    - insomnia;
    - increased anxiety and restlessness;
    - sexual dysfunction.
  - TCAs:
    - drowsiness and sedation;
    - anticholinergic (dry mouth, constipation, blurred vision, urinary hesitancy);
    - postural hypotension;
    - tachycardia and palpitations;
    - weight gain.
- Explain dosage and timing – generally TCAs at night and SSRIs in the morning.

A2: Are there other options available if he refuses?

- Mild or moderate depressive episodes respond as well to cognitive therapy as to antidepressants, though it may take longer. Cognitive therapy hypothesizes that low mood is maintained by depressive cognitions, relating to the world, the self and the future. These automatic thoughts can be targeted and alleviated, resulting in lifting of mood. Cognitive strategies can be applied in weekly 1-hour sessions over 6–10 weeks.
- Other psychological strategies such as problem-solving therapy, lifestyle management, avoidance of exacerbating factors (such as stresses or alcohol misuse) and anxiety management may be useful.

REVISION PANEL

- Mood disorders are characterized by episodes of persistent and severe elevation or depression of mood. A depressive episode is characterized by low mood, lack of energy (anergia), and a lack of interest in normal activities (anhedonia), while the key features of a manic episode are elevation of mood and increased energy or overactivity.
- Mood disorders are best thought of as biological disorders with a strong genetic component, which are often precipitated by environmental events and modified by personality traits and natural coping styles.
- Careful assessment of thoughts of self-harm and suicide is important in cases of mood disorder.
- Treatment strategies involve medication (antidepressants, mood stabilizers) and psychological interventions (cognitive behavioural therapy).
- Response to treatment should be anticipated, although recurrence of both depressive and manic episodes is likely across the lifespan.

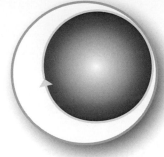

3 Anxiety disorders

Questions

Clinical cases

For each of the case scenarios given, consider the following:

> **Q1**: What is the likely differential diagnosis?
> **Q2**: What information in the history supports the diagnosis, and what other information would help to confirm it?
> **Q3**: What might the important aetiological factors be?
> **Q4**: What treatment options are available?
> **Q5**: What is the prognosis in this case?

CASE 3.1 – Anxiety associated with leaving home

A 36-year-old teacher is referred to a community mental health team by her general practitioner (GP). She is worried about her physical health, but physical examination and other tests by her GP have found no abnormalities. She describes episodes where her heart pounds, she feels hot and faint, and has an overwhelming need to escape. This first happened during a staff meeting at school, and again while in a large supermarket. Now she is apprehensive about going out in case she experiences another attack.

CASE 3.2 – Anxiety and shyness in social situations

A 29-year-old woman complains of feeling anxious while at work. Since adolescence she has been worried about speaking in front of others, worrying that she would start sweating profusely and look stupid. She tends to avoid socializing with friends and travelling in other people's cars. She has only worked intermittently over the past 10 years because every time she has a job, she resigns after working for some time as she finds it difficult working effectively with other people. Her longest period of employment was as a cleaning woman for an office block, when she would only start work after the office workers had gone home. In social situations she tends to drink too much alcohol in an effort to relax, and feels that on occasion she might have made a fool of herself.

CASE 3.3 – Unpleasant repetitive thoughts leading to unusual repetitive behaviour

A 26-year-old woman presented after her cleaning rituals had so exhausted her that she had given up and could now enter only two of the five rooms in her flat. For more than a year she has worried that if her house is not sufficiently clean, her young son will become ill and could die. Having touched a surface she has to disinfect it repeatedly – a procedure performed in a particular way and taking several hours. In addition, she repetitively washes her hands and sterilizes all the crockery and cutlery before eating. She realizes that she is 'going over the top', but she cannot stop thinking that items may have germs on them. This leads to disabling anxiety and fear for her son's health, which she can only resolve by cleaning. This helps temporarily, but soon the thoughts return again.

CASE 3.4 – **Low mood and anxiety after a very stressful event**

A 22-year-old bank clerk was involved in a severe car crash. He witnessed the death of a young woman and he had to be cut out of his car while it was on fire. He sustained only minor injuries and was able to return to work a few days later. After about 1 month he became increasingly irritable, low in mood, and anxious. He felt guilt about the death, and believed that he could have saved the woman if he had acted quicker. He could not drive near the scene of the accident without becoming extremely anxious. He could not understand why he was not coping when he had survived the accident virtually unharmed.

👥 OSCE counselling cases

OSCE COUNSELLING CASE 3.1

You have assessed a young man and made a diagnosis of panic attacks. The man is convinced that he is going to die during the attacks because of his physical symptoms.

Q1: How would you explain to this patient why his physical symptoms occur?

Key concepts

Anxiety is a normal physiological and psychological phenomenon. Everyone is familiar with the symptoms (see Table 3.1).

Table 3.1 Symptoms of anxiety

Mood	Fearfulness, apprehension	
Thoughts	Unrealistic appraisal of danger/illness to self or others	
	Lack of belief in ability to cope with stress	
Increased arousal	Difficulty sleeping	
	Restlessness and irritability	
	Noise sensitivity	
	Increased startle response	
Somatic symptoms	Hyperventilation:	Faintness, paraesthesia, carpopedal spasm
	Muscular tension:	Fatigue, pain, stiffness, tremor, chest tightness
	Autonomic overactivity:	Tachycardia, palpitation, flushing, dry mouth, diarrhoea, urinary frequency, sweating
Behaviour	Reduced purposeful activity	
	Restless purposeless activity	
	Avoidance of situations which exacerbate anxiety	

WHEN IS ANXIETY PATHOLOGICAL?

Three factors may suggest that anxiety is pathological:

- Degree – if the anxiety is far greater than most people experience.
- Situation – if the precipitant would not normally be anxiety provoking, for example insects or leaving the house.
- Consequences – if the anxiety has negative consequences or is disabling in some way, perhaps affecting an individuals functioning:
  - at work;
  - in the home;
  - in their interpersonal relationships.

DIAGNOSIS OF ANXIETY DISORDERS

The symptom of anxiety is the same in all the anxiety disorders. Diagnosis depends on the identification of associated symptoms and recognition of the appropriate syndrome. The flow chart shown in Figure 3.1 provides a simple diagnostic scheme.

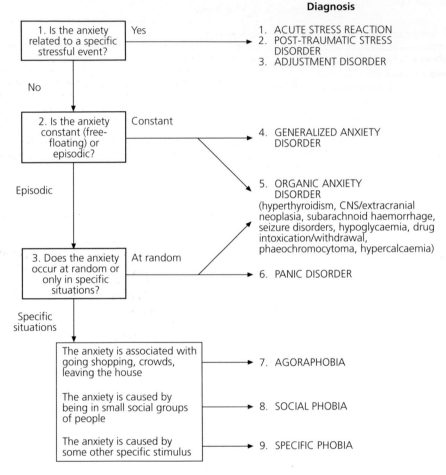

Figure 3.1 Diagnostic flow chart for anxiety disorders.

Obsessive–compulsive disorder (OCD) tends to be considered with this group because anxiety is usually a feature of the disorder.

TREATMENT OF ANXIETY DISORDERS

There are many pharmacological and psychological treatments for anxiety. Some are diagnostically non-specific, and may be used in any disorder in which anxiety is a feature. Some are used specifically for a particular diagnosis (see Table 3.2).

Table 3.2 Non-specific and diagnosis-specific psychological treatments of anxiety

Non-specific psychological treatments of anxiety	Supportive psychotherapy	
	Relaxation training	
	Problem-solving therapy	
	Anxiety management	
Diagnosis-specific psychological treatments of anxiety	Phobic anxiety disorders	Graded exposure
	Obsessive–compulsive disorder	Exposure and response prevention
		Thought stopping

For all anxiety disorders, attempts by the patient to avoid experiencing anxiety maintain the disorder. Psychological treatment depends on exposing the patient to his or her anxiety, enabling them to experience it and, over time, habituate to it.

Answers

Clinical cases

CASE 3.1 – **Anxiety associated with leaving home**

A1: What is the likely differential diagnosis?

Preferred diagnosis:

- Agoraphobia.

Alternative diagnoses:

- Panic disorder.
- Hypochondriasis.
- Depression.
- Organic anxiety disorder.

A2: What information in the history supports the diagnosis, and what other information would help to confirm it?

This woman is describing panic attacks, which are sudden, unprovoked episodes of anxiety that usually peak within a few minutes and last less than 1 hour. Physical symptoms include palpitations, sweating, shaking, shortness of breath and feeling dizzy. Such attacks are accompanied by a sense of dread, and feelings of going mad, losing control or dying.

- The apparent association of the panic attacks with leaving home and her consequent avoidance of leaving home is suggestive of agoraphobia. Further history needs to concentrate on clarifying this association.
- If the symptoms were not associated with a fear of leaving home and instead occurred at random, then the diagnosis would be panic disorder. In practice, the two disorders often occur together.
- Her worry about her health may suggest hypochondriasis, but this does not seem to be the primary problem. The history suggests that if her episodic anxiety is resolved then she will no longer have any concerns about her health.
- Anxiety symptoms are common in depression, which must be excluded by demonstrating the absence of the symptoms of a depressive syndrome.
- The normal physical examination and investigations by the GP will have ruled out an organic cause of the symptoms.

A3: What might the important aetiological factors be?

PREDISPOSING FACTORS

People with anxious personality traits may be more prone to developing the disorder. Genetic factors seem to determine an increased risk of anxiety disorders in general, rather than of agoraphobia or panic disorder specifically.

PRECIPITATING FACTORS

The episode may have been precipitated by a life event or stressor.

MAINTAINING FACTORS

Ongoing stresses or problems may be important. A further maintaining factor in phobias is avoidance of the anxiety-provoking situation. The reduction in anxiety associated with avoidance is a strong positive reinforcement for further avoidant behaviour.

A4: What treatment options are available?

LOCATION

- This case will almost certainly be treated as an outpatient.
- There is no strong relationship between agoraphobia or panic disorder and self-harm (unless there is a comorbid depressive syndrome).
- The behavioural treatment for agoraphobia is likely to be more effective in the home environment.

PHYSICAL

- A variety of antidepressants, including tricyclic antidepressants (TCAs) and the selective serotonin reuptake inhibitors (SSRIs), have been tried in agoraphobia with limited success. Up to 4 weeks of treatment is required before symptoms significantly improve.
- Benzodiazepines may be useful in the acute period for rapid symptom relief, but their effect diminishes with time and they carry the risk of dependence.
- β-Blockers may be useful in attenuating the physical symptoms of anxiety.
- If the diagnosis were panic disorder, then the first-line treatment would be a serotonergic antidepressant. These are a very effective treatment for panic disorder, with the usual caveats about delay in treatment response.

PSYCHOLOGICAL

- Simple attempts at education about anxiety and lifestyle modification (such as reduction of caffeine) may be helpful in reducing symptom severity.
- The patient should be discouraged from avoiding their anxiety-provoking situation, as the reduction in anxiety produced by avoidance will tend to maintain and exacerbate the disorder.
- The definitive treatment of agoraphobia is graded exposure, whereby the patient is exposed sequentially to a hierarchy of anxiety provoking situations and encouraged to remain at each stage until their anxiety has dissipated. This is supported by relaxation training and cognitive therapy.

A5: What is the prognosis in this case?

- The prognosis is better in the presence of comorbid depression (as this can be readily treated), a normal premorbid personality or a recent onset.
- It is not uncommon for agoraphobia to become chronic and very disabling.

CASE 3.2 – **Anxiety and shyness in social situations**

A1: What is the likely differential diagnosis?

Preferred diagnosis:

- Social phobia.

Alternative diagnoses:

- Personality disorder – probably anxious personality disorder.
- Depressive episode.
- Panic disorder.

A2: What information in the history supports the diagnosis, and what other information would help to confirm it?

The onset in adolescence of anxiety which is specifically related to social situations in which she may be under the scrutiny of other people is characteristic of social phobia, as is the overvalued idea that she may sweat or humiliate herself. Alcohol is a common way for people to relax socially, and alcohol misuse commonly complicates social phobia.

- An onset in adolescence may also suggest personality disorder. Anxious personality disorder is characterized by persistent feelings of tension, a belief that one is socially inept or inferior to others, a preoccupation with being criticized and avoidance of social activities that require interpersonal contact. Anxious personality disorder and social phobia are very similar and often coexist.
- Depression may exacerbate pre-existing anxious personality traits and should be excluded as it is readily treatable.
- You must be sure that the episodes of anxiety are specifically related to social situations. If they occur at other times too, then panic disorder may be the most appropriate diagnosis.

A3: What might the important aetiological factors be?

PREDISPOSING FACTORS

Social phobia may be more likely in people with anxious personality traits.

PRECIPITATING FACTORS

Life stressors or problems may precipitate and exacerbate the disorder.

MAINTAINING FACTORS

Alcohol or substance misuse is common. Avoidance of the anxiety-provoking situation is also a maintaining factor, as the reduction in anxiety associated with avoidance is a strong positive reinforcement for further avoidant behaviour.

A4: What treatment options are available?

LOCATION

This case will almost certainly be treated as an outpatient unless there is also a risk of self-harm.

PHYSICAL

- Some serotonergic antidepressants are licensed for the treatment of social phobia. They are more likely to be effective in the presence of symptoms of depression.
- Benzodiazepines have little role because social phobia is usually a long-standing disorder that is likely to take some time to treat.
- β-Blockers could be used prophylactically for specific predictable situations. However, these are unlikely to have much effect on the overvalued ideas relating to social humiliation that drive the anxiety.

PSYCHOLOGICAL

The diagnosis non-specific treatments can all be used.

SOCIAL

- Social skills or assertiveness training may be useful for a patient who is particularly shy or lacking in self-esteem.
- Cognitive therapy reduces the overvalued ideas of social humiliation.

A5: What is the prognosis in this case?

- Symptoms of social phobia are very common in adolescence, but usually wane as the person enters adulthood.
- The prognosis is better in the presence of comorbid depression (which can be easily treated) and worse the more the social phobia resembles a personality disorder (personality disorders are chronic by definition).

CASE 3.3 – **Unpleasant repetitive thoughts leading to unusual repetitive behaviour**

A1: What is the likely differential diagnosis?

Preferred diagnosis:

- Obsessive–compulsive disorder.

Alternative diagnoses:

- Depressive disorder.
- Schizophrenia.
- Anankastic personality disorder.

A2: What information in the history supports the diagnosis, and what other information would help to confirm it?

This history clearly describes obsessions and compulsions, but further history-taking should clarify the essential features. Obsessions are repetitive, intrusive and stereotyped thoughts, images or impulses. The patient knows they are irrational or silly and tries to resist them, but they are recognized as the patient's own. Compulsions are voluntary actions which the patient performs in order to reduce the build up of anxiety and tension caused by the obsession. There may be a family history of OCD or other anxiety disorders.

- The history should always exclude a depressive episode, which may sometimes present with obsessions and compulsions.
- Schizophrenia should be considered for two reasons:
  - obsessional symptoms are common in the early stages of schizophrenia, before a person has developed frank psychosis;
  - repetitive intrusive thoughts may suggest thought insertion (first rank symptom of schizophrenia), so it is important to ensure that the patient recognizes the thought as their own.
- Someone with anankastic personality disorder is excessively cautious and unwilling to take risks, and is preoccupied with rules and details. A high level of perfectionism prevents them from completing tasks, and they may be pedantic and stubborn. Insistent or unwelcome thoughts or impulses come into their mind in a similar way to obsessions, but the characteristic coupling of severe obsessions and compulsions described above would not occur. People with anankastic personality disorder may develop OCD and are at an increased risk of developing depressive episodes.

A3: What might the important aetiological factors be?

PREDISPOSING FACTORS

A family history of OCD is a predisposing factor, though it is not certain that this is genetically mediated.

PRECIPITATING FACTORS

Stressful life events are common precipitating factors.

MAINTAINING FACTORS

Ongoing stresses or problems may be important. A further perpetuating factor is the compulsion itself. The reduction of anxiety that results from performing the compulsion provides a strong positive reinforcement and makes the same behaviour more likely in the future. This is analogous to the maintaining effect of avoidance in phobic disorders.

A4: What treatment options are available?

LOCATION

- Treatment of OCD is usually undertaken on an outpatient basis. In some very severe or resistant cases admission to hospital may become necessary to allow more intensive treatment and closer support and monitoring.
- Comorbid depression may also necessitate admission.

PHYSICAL

- Serotonergic antidepressants (clomipramine or selective serotonin reuptake inhibitors [SSRIs] are effective when used in higher doses than are necessary in depression.
- In severe cases, benzodiazepines may be useful in the short term to reduce anxiety that is preventing the patients from engaging in behavioural treatments.
- For the most intractable and severe cases, psychosurgery (limbic leucotomy) may be considered.

PSYCHOLOGICAL

- The first step in treatment is to explain to the patient the way in which continued compulsive behaviour perpetuates the disorder. Preventing this is the mainstay of psychological treatment, a technique called exposure and response prevention. This aims to support the patient in not performing their compulsive rituals and tolerating the consequent anxiety, for increasingly long periods of time. Adjunctive relaxation training and cognitive therapy may help with toleration of the anxiety.
- In the rare cases where obsessions exist in the absence of compulsions, thought stopping may be used.

A5: What is the prognosis in this case?

- The course of OCD is variable. It is common for the disorder to be persistent, though improved by treatment. A phasic course is common, with exacerbations of severity at stressful times in life, followed by relative quiescence when the patient's life is more stable or settled.
- If it is associated with depressive symptoms, the prognosis is improved (because depression is readily treatable), while the prognosis is worse in the presence of abnormal personality traits.

CASE 3.4 – **Low mood and anxiety after a very stressful event**

A1: What is the likely differential diagnosis?

Preferred diagnosis:

- Post-traumatic stress disorder (PTSD).

Alternative diagnoses:

- Acute stress disorder.
- Adjustment disorder.
- Depression.
- Panic disorder.
- Generalized anxiety disorder.

A2: What information in the history supports the diagnosis, and what other information would help to confirm it?

The patient is complaining of symptoms of anxiety specifically related to a particularly stressful event. The history should look for the triad of re-experiencing symptoms (intrusive thoughts/memories, nightmares or flashbacks), hypervigilance (difficulty sleeping, enhanced startle reflex, autonomic overactivity, irritability and reduced concentration) and avoidance behaviour (reduced emotional responsiveness, lack of pleasure, restlessness, avoiding situations reminiscent of the event, increased fantasy life). In addition, the common associated features of depression and alcohol/substance misuse should be excluded.

- The onset is delayed, which suggests PTSD and excludes an acute stress reaction.
- An adjustment disorder is a psychological reaction to a significant change in life circumstances rather than to a specific stressful event. It is mild in severity and rarely requires psychiatric treatment.
- If low mood and a depressive syndrome are prominent, depression is the more appropriate diagnosis.
- If the anxiety was not related specifically to the car crash, then panic disorder (if it is episodic) or generalized anxiety disorder (if it is constant) may be more appropriate diagnoses.

A3: What might the important aetiological factors be?

PREDISPOSING FACTORS

An individual may be predisposed to develop PTSD by a personal or family history of mild depressive illness, anxiety disorders or abnormal personality traits.

PRECIPITATING FACTORS

The essential precipitating factor is an exceptionally stressful life event, in this case the car crash. The PTSD, by definition, would not have occurred without it.

MAINTAINING FACTORS

Maintaining factors may include avoidance (as with phobias), and maladaptive coping strategies such as alcohol or substance misuse.

A4: What treatment options are available?

LOCATION

This is most likely to occur as an outpatient, though if very severe, or associated with a depressive episode or a significant risk of self-harm, admission may be considered.

PHYSICAL

- Serotonergic antidepressants are claimed to be useful by some, though response is predicted by the presence of depressive symptoms. Therefore, the primary treatment effect may be antidepressant.
- Benzodiazepines should be avoided because of the risk of dependence with prolonged use.

PSYCHOLOGICAL

- A variety of different approaches have been used, from supportive psychotherapy to more formal cognitive techniques and dynamic psychotherapy.
- It seems that the important feature is that the treatment takes place in a group setting, providing the patient with support from others who are experiencing similar problems.

A5: What is the prognosis in this case?

- It is important for treatment to be instituted promptly. Once PTSD is long-standing and maladaptive coping strategies are ingrained, it is likely to become chronic and potentially disabling. The prognosis is also worse in those with a history of psychiatric disorder, abnormal premorbid personality and poor social support.

● It is worth noting that 'debriefing' people immediately after a stressful event does not prevent – and probably increases – the likelihood of developing PTSD. It may be useful to identify those at particular risk (intense acute reaction to event, previous psychiatric history, particularly direct involvement in event) and to counsel them, but this should not be done indiscriminately.

♀♂ OSCE counselling cases

OSCE COUNSELLING CASE 3.1

You have assessed a young man and made a diagnosis of panic attacks. The man is convinced that he is going to die during the attacks because of his physical symptoms.

A1: How would you explain to this patient why his physical symptoms occur?

- It may be helpful to draw a diagram linking his thoughts (cognitions) with his anxiety (feelings) with his physical symptoms and back to his cognitions (see Figure 3.2).

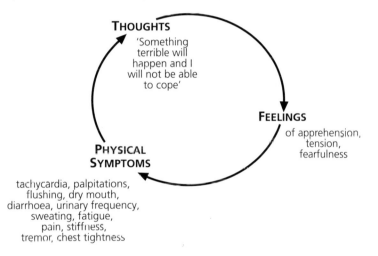

THOUGHTS
'Something terrible will happen and I will not be able to cope'

FEELINGS
of apprehension, tension, fearfulness

PHYSICAL SYMPTOMS
tachycardia, palpitations, flushing, dry mouth, diarrhoea, urinary frequency, sweating, fatigue, pain, stiffness, tremor, chest tightness

Figure 3.2 A vicious circle of anxiety.

- Identifying the cognitions that precede an attack may be difficult, but a careful history going through a specific attack in detail or thought diaries can help.
- Careful description of all the physical symptoms with suggestions from you of what they may be can help the patient to believe that they are symptomatic of anxiety rather than a physical illness. Explanation of the physiology (fright, fight and flight) of panic can help the patient to understand how thoughts and feelings can result in physical symptoms.
- Discuss how experiencing these symptoms can lead to further catastrophic cognitions and increased levels of anxiety. This is often thought of as a vicious circle.
- Two experiments can be used to link the different elements of the cycle. First, hyperventilation can induce feelings of anxiety. Second, thinking about the thoughts and situations in which panic attacks occur may induce symptoms of a panic attack.
- Once the patient understands and believes this cycle, work can begin to break it at various different points.

REVISION PANEL

- Anxiety is a normal human response to certain situations. Pathological anxiety is distinguished by its degree, the precipitating situation and its consequences.
- Antidepressants are effective anxiolytics. They are most likely to be effective in acute mental illnesses, particularly panic disorder.
- Long-standing generalized anxiety is likely to respond less well to pharmacological treatment and tends to follow a waxing and waning course.
- Psychological treatment of anxiety disorders necessarily requires exposure of the patient to their anxiety, in a graduated and supportive way, allowing them to habituate to it.

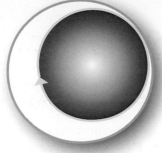

4 Chronic disorders

Questions

Clinical cases

For each of the case scenarios given, consider the following:

> **Q1**: What pharmacological strategies are available?
> **Q2**: What psychological strategies are available?
> **Q3**: What social factors are important?

CASE 4.1 – **Persistent symptoms of psychosis in schizophrenia**

A 38-year-old man has had schizophrenia for many years. He has been admitted to hospital repeatedly during episodes of acute psychosis. These symptoms initially responded to treatment with medication, but over recent years the symptoms have become increasingly persistent and resistant. He has had trials of a variety of antipsychotic medications, including depot preparations.

He is now in hospital recovering from an episode of acute illness. Although he has improved since he was admitted, he continues to experience persistent auditory hallucinations. These take the form of commentary auditory hallucinations and voices in the third person insulting him. He understands that they are caused by his illness, but when he experiences them he nonetheless finds them very distressing and intrusive.

CASE 4.2 – **Poor motivation, apathy and social isolation in schizophrenia**

A 50-year-old man was diagnosed with schizophrenia at the age of 27. In the intervening years he has had many admissions due to recurrent psychotic episodes. Negative symptoms became evident early in the course of his illness and have steadily deteriorated.

He lives with his elderly parents, but has an impoverished life, with few hobbies, pastimes or social outlets. His self-care and hygiene are poor, and he spends most of his time watching television alone in his room. He is compliant with his maintenance depot antipsychotic medication, which is administered by his community psychiatric nurse.

He has continued to have occasional episodes of psychosis requiring inpatient admission.

CASE 4.3 – **Repeated episodes of mania**

A 32-year-old man was admitted under Section 3 of the Mental Health Act 1983 with his second episode of mania. The episode began with difficulty sleeping and restlessness during the day. He described his thoughts racing, and at the time of admission he had grandiose delusions and flight of ideas. His symptoms responded well to antipsychotic treatment, and 2 weeks after admission, plans were being made for his longer-term management.

⁂ OSCE counselling cases

OSCE COUNSELLING CASE 4.1

A 45-year-old man is referred to a psychiatric outpatient clinic by his GP. He developed the symptoms of a depressive episode 2 months before the referral, including low mood and tearfulness, a loss of energy, decreased motivation and suicidal thoughts. His GP started him on fluoxetine (a selective serotonin reuptake inhibitor) at a dose of 20 mg per day 5 weeks prior to the appointment with the psychiatrist, but he feels no better.

Q1: Describe how you would treat this man pharmacologically if his depression continues without improvement.

Q2: What psychological strategies might be helpful?

🔑 Key concepts

Good psychiatric practice emphasizes early detection and intervention, a focus on long-term recovery and promoting people's choices about the management of their condition. There is evidence that most people will recover, although many disorders encountered by psychiatrists run a chronic course. Chronicity has two important aspects:

- Some disorders persist, despite appropriate treatment. For example, negative symptoms of schizophrenia respond poorly to medical management.
- Some disorders are episodic; for example, a person may have acute episodes of mania or depression in bipolar disorder throughout their entire life.

In all cases, the following steps should be regularly considered:

- Review the diagnosis and consider treating comorbid conditions such as substance misuse.
- Check the patient's compliance with treatment and review their medication history.
- Consider maintaining factors – psychosocial stressors, family influences, coping abilities, physical illness, drug misuse.

In the longer term, most people will find ways to manage acute problems, and compensate for any remaining difficulties. Carers, relatives and friends of people with chronic mental illness are important in the successful long-term delivery of effective treatments.

Other key principles to bear in mind are:

- Treatment should always take into account the patient's needs and preferences.
- Patients should have the opportunity to make informed decisions, including advance decisions and advance statements, about their care and treatment, in partnership with their doctor and healthcare professionals.
- If patients do not have the capacity to make decisions, healthcare professionals should follow guidance outlined in the Mental Capacity Act.
- Good communication between doctors and their patients is essential, ideally supported by evidence-based written information tailored to the patient's needs.
- All aspects of care, and the information patients and their carers are given about it, should be culturally appropriate. It should also be accessible to people with additional needs such as physical, sensory or learning disabilities, and to people who do not speak or read English.

PHYSICAL HEALTH AND CHRONIC PSYCHIATRIC DISORDERS

People with schizophrenia or bipolar disorder have higher levels of physical morbidity and mortality than the general population, but may receive suboptimal healthcare. Those at increased risk of developing cardiovascular disease and/or diabetes (for example, with elevated blood pressure, raised lipid levels, smokers, increased waist measurement) should be identified as early as possible.

Key elements of the initial assessment include:

- Recording the patient's smoking status and alcohol use.
- Full blood count (FBC), blood glucose, lipid profile, thyroid function tests, liver function tests (LFTs) and urea and electrolytes (U&Es).
- Weight, height and blood pressure measurement.
- Electroencephalography (EEG), computed tomography (CT) or magnetic resonance imaging (MRI) if an organic aetiology or a relevant comorbidity is suspected.
- Drug screening, chest X-ray and electrocardiography (ECG) if suggested by the history or clinical picture.

On-going monitoring during long-term treatment is also important. This may require good coordination between primary care and secondary mental health services.

- Medication used to treat chronic psychiatric disorders can result in significant weight gain. Patients taking antipsychotics should have their weight checked every 3 months for the first year, and more often if they gain weight rapidly.
- Plasma glucose and lipids (preferably fasting levels) should be measured 3 months after the start of treatment and more often if there is evidence of elevated levels.
- The patient should be aware of the risk of weight gain, and the possibility of worsening existing diabetes, malignant neuroleptic syndrome and diabetic ketoacidosis with the use of antipsychotic medication.

An annual physical health review, normally in primary care, should include:

- Lipid levels, including cholesterol in all patients over 40.
- Plasma glucose levels.
- Weight and blood pressure measurement.
- Smoking status and alcohol use assessment.

The results of the annual review should be given to the patient, and a clear agreement should be made between primary and secondary care about responsibility for treating any problems.

If a person gains weight during treatment their medication should be reviewed, and the following considered:

- Dietary advice and support from primary care and mental health services.
- Advising regular aerobic exercise.
- Referral for specific programmes to manage weight gain.
- Referral to a dietician if the person has complex comorbidities (e.g. coeliac disease).

Answers

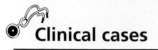

Clinical cases

CASE 4.1 – **Persistent symptoms of psychosis in schizophrenia**

A1: What pharmacological strategies are available?

- If compliance is poor – and particularly if it is due to disorganization or forgetfulness rather than active refusal – a depot antipsychotic might be considered.
- Pharmacological management of treatment-resistant schizophrenia:
  - trial of an adequate dose of one antipsychotic for at least 6 weeks;
  - trial of an adequate dose of a second antipsychotic for at least 6 weeks (at least one of these two medications should be an atypical antipsychotic);
  - trial of clozapine at an adequate dose; ideally, this should be assessed over at least 6 months as some patients show a delayed response.

No other pharmacological strategy has a clear evidence base. Options to consider include combining clozapine with another antipsychotic, high doses of some antipsychotics, addition of lithium or other mood stabilizers or omega-3-triglycerides.

- Clozapine is the only antipsychotic that has been shown unequivocally to be more effective than the other antipsychotics in treatment-resistant patients. However, it is associated with an increased rate of agranulocytosis. Therefore it can only be prescribed on a named-patient basis, and the neutrophil count must be monitored weekly initially, subsequently reducing to monthly for the duration of treatment.
- Unproven therapies should be carefully evaluated in individual patients, preferably with recognized symptom scales.

A2: What psychological strategies are available?

- If compliance with medication is poor, adherence therapy techniques may be considered. These provide education about mental illness, medication and the importance of compliance for treatment to be effective.
- Consider maintaining factors such as substance misuse, and educate the patient about their negative effect on treatment response.
- Cognitive behavioural therapy (CBT) is now recommended for all people with schizophrenia. This is usually delivered on a one-to-one basis, following a treatment manual. It aims to help the patient establish links between their thoughts, feelings, or actions and their current and/or past symptoms and experiences, and to re-evaluate these connections. The overall aim is to reduce distress and improve functioning.
- Behavioural strategies used for auditory hallucinations include distraction techniques such as listening to music/watching television, sub-vocal counting, talking back to the voices, actively listening to them for a specific period each day and ignoring them the rest of the time. The success of these tends to be idiosyncratic, so the patient should be encouraged to try out different things.
- Delusions may be targeted using cognitive therapy in a similar way to other thoughts.

Finally, always remember that any symptom may be exacerbated by subjective stress or anxiety. Therefore, strategies such as relaxation training, anxiety management and problem-solving therapy may be useful in particular patients.

A3: What social factors are important?

- Financial worries, poor housing, difficult interpersonal relationships, and poor social networks may all contribute to subjective stress and thereby exacerbate persistent psychotic symptoms.
- Occupational activities should be considered. It is important not to make too many demands on a patient who has persistent psychotic symptoms.

CASE 4.2 – **Poor motivation, apathy and social isolation in schizophrenia**

A1: What pharmacological strategies are available?

- Negative symptoms of schizophrenia generally respond poorly to medication. In fact, they are often exacerbated by the sedating effect of antipsychotics, particularly typical antipsychotics. Therefore, one pharmacological approach would be to replace his depot medication with an atypical oral antipsychotic. It would be important to prepare him for this, and to consider how you will promote compliance.
- The only antipsychotic that has proven efficacy in treating negative symptoms is clozapine. Therefore, this might also be considered and may also be of benefit in reducing the likelihood of relapse.

A2: What psychological strategies are available?

- The management of chronic schizophrenia needs to strike a balance between under-stimulation and over-stimulation.
- Episodes of psychosis are known to be associated with stress or over-stimulation. It may be that negative symptoms are in part a mechanism to reduce the impact of such stress. Social withdrawal and lack of activity may reduce the demands placed on the patient and thereby help to protect against the emergence of psychosis.
- However, an under-stimulating environment may promote negative symptoms, which themselves may be disabling for the patient.
- One particular stressor that has been shown to be associated with an increased rate of relapse of psychosis is expressed emotion. This is defined as the level of critical comments, over-involved attitude and intrusive behaviour displayed by the patient's carers. Family therapy is a psychological strategy that aims to reduce this by promoting understanding and empathy among carers.
- Family therapy should include the person with schizophrenia if possible, and usually involves 10 or more planned and structured sessions over 3–12 months. They have a specific supportive, educational or treatment function and include negotiated problem solving or crisis management work.
- If family therapy is not possible, an alternative approach is to reduce the amount of time that the patient is in contact with his or her carers. This may entail finding alternative accommodation, or providing day care.

Participation in a group run by an experienced arts therapist may also be beneficial. Arts therapies combine psychotherapeutic techniques with activity aimed at promoting creative expression, which is often unstructured and led by the patient. They aim to enable people with schizophrenia to experience themselves differently and to develop new ways of relating to others, while also helping them to accept and understand feelings that may have emerged during the creative process.

A3: What social factors are important?

- The provision of day care may be helpful in providing structure and motivation in a patient's life, reducing the amount of time spent in contact with high expressed emotion, and improving social networks as well as facilitating monitoring of mental state.

- Areas to consider include:
  - functional assessment and training in activities of daily living such as cooking, budgeting and personal care;
  - employment and occupational training;
  - social skills training;
  - problem-solving therapy.
- Respite care in hospital may provide some families with regular breaks from the stress of caring for a patient with severe and enduring illness. This can help reduce the expressed emotion within the family.

CASE 4.3 – **Repeated episodes of mania**

A1: What pharmacological strategies are available?

After two episodes of mania, prophylaxis with a mood stabilizer is necessary to prevent recurrence of mania (or depression). The best known of these drugs is lithium:

- Baseline height, weight, FBC, U&Es, TFTs, and ECG for patients at risk of cardiovascular disease, are required prior to starting treatment.
- Lithium is usually started at a low dose (200–400 mg nocte), and the levels checked 12 h after the last dose in 5–7 days' time. If the blood levels are below the therapeutic range, the dose should be increased and the monitoring process repeated.
- Once a patient is stabilized then lithium levels are monitored at least 3 monthly; TFTs and renal function are monitored 6 monthly.
- The therapeutic range of lithium is narrow, so close monitoring of the plasma concentration is essential. A plasma concentration between 0.4 and 1.0 mmol/L is required for prophylaxis, with doses at the upper end of this range needed for acute treatment. Symptoms of lithium toxicity begin to appear at serum concentrations above 2.5 mmol/L.
- The benefits, risks, side effects (see Table 4.1) and monitoring must be discussed with the patient and their carers.
- The patient should be warned of the dangers of dehydration, as this may lead to the kidneys retaining lithium and producing toxic levels. It is best to try to drink plenty of fluids and to stop the lithium and seek medical advice in the case of severe vomiting or diarrhoea. Careful consideration needs to be given to starting lithium in women of childbearing age, as the drug is teratogenic.

Alternative mood stabilizers include the anticonvulsants valproate, carbamazepine and lamotrigine, and the atypical antipsychotics (aripiprazole, quetiapine and olanzapine, in particular). The choice of medication will depend on which treatment the patient was receiving prior to the manic episode, previous response to treatment, the potential side effect profile, and patient choice. The available medicines appear to be more effective against one pole of the illness than the other, with lithium and the antipsychotics being more effective against manic relapse.

Table 4.1 Side effects and toxic effects of lithium therapy

Side effects	Dry mouth with a metallic taste
	Thirst
	Mild polyuria
	Nausea
	Weight gain
	Fine tremor of the hands
	Hypothyroidism (in approximately 20%)
	Renal impairment may be associated with long-term use
Symptoms of toxicity (start to appear at concentrations >2.5 mmol/L)	Increasing thirst and polyuria
	Coarse tremor
	Agitation
	Twitching
	Myoclonic jerks
	Renal failure
	Seizures
	Coma
	Death

A2: What psychological strategies are available?

- A fundamental aim of the treatment of bipolar disorder is to educate the patient in order to improve their ability to evaluate the risks posed to them by the illness.
- Non-compliance with medication is a serious problem. Concerns over side effects, or a dislike for taking medication when otherwise well, are understandable, and require careful consideration by the prescribing doctor. 'Motivational enhancement' strategies have been shown to be effective at increasing medication compliance in this group.
- The onset of a manic episode usually progresses through identifiable stages that occur over a number of hours to days. These are often consistent for individual patients. Being aware of the early warning signs (called a 'relapse signature') and acting immediately has been shown to decrease the potential severity and duration of the episode. These symptoms may include increased activity, decreased need for sleep, irritability or elated mood. Therapeutic strategies involve training the patient to identify such prodromal symptoms, and then producing and rehearsing an action plan to deal with them.
- CBT may be helpful in tackling depressive episodes in the context of a bipolar affective disorder.
- Family-focused therapy consisting of psychoeducation about bipolar disorder, communication enhancement training, and problem-solving skills training has also been shown to be beneficial.

A3: What social factors are important?

- An acute manic episode can lead to the accumulation of a variety of social problems. The patient may regret their previous actions when their mental state returns to normal, and need supportive work to overcome the distress that their behaviour may have caused.
- Large debts can often be run up during a grandiose period, and debt advisers may be able to help the patient deal with this effectively.
- Considerable work may be necessary to support carers and to rebuild their confidence in looking after the patient. Social factors such as poor housing, social isolation and unemployment may be a source of stress, and precipitate future recurrence.
- Patients with chronic, relapsing disorders such as bipolar affective disorder often benefit from 'case management'. This means that a member of the multidisciplinary mental health team is designated

the 'key worker' and will draw up a plan of care in conjunction with the patient and their carers. This may include actions to be taken in the event of a relapse of the illness, and will be regularly reviewed. This can enable the patient and their carers to access effective treatment and support at an early stage, thus preventing a more serious and prolonged bout of illness.

⚇ OSCE counselling cases

OSCE COUNSELLING CASE 4.1

A 45-year-old man is referred to a psychiatric outpatient clinic by his GP. He developed the symptoms of a depressive episode 2 months before the referral, including low mood and tearfulness, a loss of energy, decreased motivation and suicidal thoughts. His GP started him on fluoxetine (a selective serotonin reuptake inhibitor) at a dose of 20 mg per day 5 weeks prior to the appointment with the psychiatrist, but he feels no better.

A1: Describe how you would treat this man pharmacologically if his depression continues without improvement.

- Review the diagnosis – depression often presents with other comorbid disorders such as panic disorder, obsessive–compulsive disorder or alcohol misuse or dependence, and these may require treatment if the depressive symptoms are to improve.
- Check compliance with prescribed dose of medication and address concerns such as fear of addiction or side effects and misunderstandings about depression or mental illness.
- Consider maintaining factors such as bereavement issues, interpersonal conflict or financial or social stressors.
- Pharmacological management of treatment-resistant depression:
  - increase dose of current antidepressant to maximum tolerated and evaluate response over 4–6 weeks;
  - change to a different class of antidepressant and evaluate over 4–6 weeks;
  - augment antidepressant with lithium and evaluate over 4 weeks;
  - augment with triiodothyronine or electroconvulsive therapy (ECT) and assess over 4 weeks or over eight sessions of ECT;
  - consider strategies with limited evidence base – high dose of antidepressants, augmentation with tryptophan, combinations of antidepressants.
- Throughout this process the patient's clinical state must be monitored closely. If a severe deterioration occurs, or there is a risk of harm to self or to others, admission to hospital may become necessary.
- If psychotic symptoms occur in depression, then combination treatment with an antidepressant and an antipsychotic is necessary.

A2: What psychological strategies might be helpful?

Psychological treatment may also benefit the patient and may augment the effect of the pharmacological treatment.

- During an episode of depression even simple problems can be difficult to solve, leading to a reinforcement of the person's already low self-esteem. Training in problem-solving techniques can counter this and so reduce helplessness.
- Behavioural therapy aims to tackle the lack of energy and enjoyment caused by depression by developing structured activity programs, rating pleasure and achievement and feeding back the results to the patient.
- Depression also tends to make people think that their problems will never improve, and leads them to a number of distorted or exaggerated thoughts. They tend to generalize problems in one area to the rest of their life, and dwell on negative events but not positive ones. Cognitive therapy therefore aims to identify and adapt such unhelpful thought patterns and, when combined with behavioural techniques, can be extremely effective.

REVISION PANEL

- Many psychiatric disorders are relapsing and remitting conditions, and sustained periods of illness are possible. Despite this it is important to retain a positive outlook, and aim to support the patient in optimizing their symptom control and day-to-day functioning.
- It is important to optimize the patient's ability to adhere to medical or psychological treatments. Good-quality education, regular consideration of patient choice, involvement of family members and carers, and regular monitoring of progress and side effects may all help.
- Incomplete response to treatment should be assessed and managed. A systematic approach to prescribing, combined with appropriate psychosocial interventions, is likely to yield the best results.

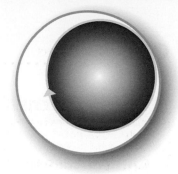

5 Older people

Questions

Clinical cases

For each of the case scenarios given, consider the following:

Q1: What is the likely differential diagnosis?
Q2: What information in the history supports the diagnosis, and what other information would help to confirm it?
Q3: What might the important aetiological factors be?
Q4: What treatment options are available?
Q5: What is the prognosis in this case?

CASE 5.1 – **Low mood and forgetfulness**

You are asked to see a 68-year-old man who lives at home with his wife, who is his sole carer. Over recent months he has been becoming increasingly forgetful. His wife comments that he begins tasks, such as making a cup of tea, and then forgets what he is doing. Two days ago he went out to buy a newspaper and came home with a tin of cat food. He is aware of this, and has been becoming increasingly worried and low in mood. His sleep is poor at night and he often gets up very early in the morning.

He has a past history of depression, having received outpatient treatment with antidepressants about 20 years ago after the death of his parents. Otherwise he has no past medical history.

CASE 5.2 – **Behavioural problems in dementia**

You are asked to see a 79-year-old man who was diagnosed with dementia 6 years previously. He lives with his 72-year-old wife. She describes a gradual deterioration in his condition such that in recent months she has found it increasingly difficult to manage him. He has become increasingly hostile and aggressive, though he has not actually assaulted her. He has begun to complain of seeing people wandering around the house, and that frightens him. On two occasions he has left the house and been found wandering along the road. She has noticed that his condition fluctuates – sometimes he is very aggressive and confused, while at other times he is more calm and lucid.

CASE 5.3 – **Persecutory ideas developing in old age**

A general practitioner (GP) asks you to perform a domiciliary visit on a 72-year-old partially deaf woman who has lived alone since the death of her husband 18 months ago. The GP says that she has always been a shy, quiet woman with little social network or support and keeps herself to herself. He visited her recently to perform an annual physical review, and she told him that she was becoming increasingly concerned about intruders entering her house at night. She had noticed that when she came downstairs each morning, furniture and ornaments had been moved around, and food in the fridge had been disturbed. She was becoming increasingly frightened that these people meant her some harm and were intending to rape or kill her. She has heard them shouting her name and can get no peace from them.

She has no psychiatric history and is relatively well physically. She has been living independently so far, with only occasional help from her children, who live some distance away.

CASE 5.4 – **Severe low mood in old age**

A 74-year-old woman, who lives alone and independently, is referred to the outpatient department. She is accompanied by her son who returned from a 3-week holiday to find her in 'a terrible state'. She seemed fine when he left, though she has always been a worrier. On his return, the son found that her house was untidy and she looked unkempt. She appeared agitated and scared. She kept following him around the house as he tried to clear up, asking him if he was going to leave her alone. He noticed that her hands were shaking and her voice trembling. She did not seem able to sit still, and was constantly pacing around the house, wringing her hands.

OSCE counselling cases

OSCE COUNSELLING CASE 5.1

You have recently diagnosed an elderly widower as having dementia. Although his cognitive function is quite severely impaired, he has expressed a wish to remain at home and you have decided to support him in this for now. His daughter asks to see you because she is very concerned about his ability to live independently. She thinks that he needs to be placed in a home.

Q1: What issues would you discuss with her?

🔑 Key concepts

Psychological problems related to increasing age include:

- Retirement, loss of occupational identity and reduced sense of self-worth.
- Loss of spouse.
- Existential concerns related to mortality.
- Reducing independence.

Physical problems related to increasing age include:

- Failing physical health and reduced mobility.
- Polypharmacy and increased sensitivity to side effects.

Social problems related to increasing age include:

- Poverty.
- Poorer accommodation.
- Poor social networks and isolation.

Therefore, assessment of the elderly has an increased focus on social problems, activities of daily living and physical health. Remember that suicide is more common with increasing age. It is also important to consider the needs of the main carer(s) and to assess their ability and desire to cope with the patient. Carer abuse is probably more common than is generally recognized.

It is important to assess the elderly patient's capacity to consent to treatment. If they do not have capacity to consent you may consider treating them under the Mental Capacity Act with Deprivation of Liberty Safeguards (DOLS). Most psychiatric disorders are broadly similar to those occurring in younger adults, but there are particular disorders characteristic of old age. Dementia and delirium are common, and should be distinguished from the amnesic syndrome:

- **Dementia** is an acquired, global impairment of cognitive function that is usually progressive. The areas which may be involved include memory (almost always), language, abstract thinking and judgement, visuospatial skills and personality. These impairments should occur without disturbance of consciousness.
- **Delirium** is a syndrome of acute onset, with fluctuating intensity that is usually worse at night. The central deficit is impaired attention and disturbed consciousness. In addition, there is a global disturbance of cognition often including perceptual illusions, misinterpretations and hallucinations and transient delusions. Psychomotor disturbance, alteration of the sleep–wake cycle and abnormal, labile mood states are also common.
- **Amnesic syndrome** is a specific deficit of new learning resulting in anterograde amnesia and disorientation in time. Immediate recall is preserved, as are attention and concentration and other cognitive functions. A variable retrograde amnesia with a temporal gradient is present, and confabulation may be marked.
- **Psychotic syndromes** occur commonly and may complicate affective illness. Late-onset schizophrenia (sometimes called paraphrenia) is a non-affective psychosis with relatively good prognosis and few negative symptoms. This may be difficult to distinguish from paranoid psychosis occurring in dementia. Persistent delusional disorders may also present in the elderly, particularly in those with a previous paranoid personality.

Answers

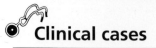

Clinical cases

CASE 5.1 – **Low mood and forgetfulness**

A1: What is the likely differential diagnosis?

Preferred diagnosis:

- Dementia.

Alternative diagnosis:

- Depressive episode.

A2: What information in the history supports the diagnosis, and what other information would help to confirm it?

Dementia is clearly suggested by this patient's gradual onset of forgetfulness. Cognitive examination should aim to test orientation, attention and concentration, registration, recall and long-term memory. Deficits in visuospatial, language and executive function skills and dyspraxia should also be assessed. In practice, you may use a screening instrument such as the Mini Mental State Examination (MMSE).

- A physical screen for reversible causes of dementia and medical conditions which can exacerbate the symptoms of dementia will include:
  - full blood count;
  - urea and electrolytes;
  - liver function tests;
  - thyroid function tests;
  - blood glucose;
  - vitamin B_{12} and folate.

Brain imaging is recommended in all age groups.

- A careful history and mental state examination (MSE) should reveal symptoms of a depressive syndrome if it is present.
- In some elderly patients, depression can present with a reversible cognitive decline (i.e. it improves as the depression is treated). This is known as 'pseudodementia'. It may be suggested clinically by a subjective awareness of cognitive decline, an acute onset, a tendency to answer questions with 'I don't know' rather than confabulate and a history, or symptoms, of affective disorder.

A3: What might the important aetiological factors be?

PREDISPOSING FACTORS

The aetiological factors associated with dementia depend on the underlying pathology, which may not be certain clinically. You need to enquire about a personal or family history of cardiovascular disease, stroke, hypertension or diabetes, which may predispose to vascular dementia. A family history of Alzheimer's dementia or other less common dementias may be important.

PRECIPITATING FACTORS

A physical illness or stressor may have led to a deterioration in his symptoms, or he may have a comorbid depressive illness which has contributed to a deterioration. Drugs such as sedatives or analgesics can precipitate a deterioration.

MAINTAINING FACTORS

Ongoing psychiatric or physical disorders should be excluded.

A4: What treatment options are available?

LOCATION
- In cases of mild dementia, investigation and management at home should be possible.
- You need to carry out a risk assessment, asking about dangerous behaviours, such as wandering, leaving the fire on, irritability and aggression and self-harm.
- You also need to consider whether his wife is coping, and what help she needs.

PHYSICAL
- In dementia due to Alzheimer's disease, cholinesterase inhibitors may delay the progression of dementia and perhaps lead to a slight improvement. There is some debate about the benefits and most appropriate use of these medications, which should be used as a part of specialist multidisciplinary care.

PSYCHOLOGICAL
- Discussion, explanation, support and reassurance are important for patients and carers. Simple memory aids such as reminder notes, alarm clocks, medication packs in daily doses may be useful.

SOCIAL
- Attendance at a day centre or day hospital provides social networks, respite for carers and an opportunity for activity, assessment and enjoyment. Help with accessing financial benefits may reduce such pressures on the family.

A5: What is the prognosis in this case?
- In the short term, improvements in his clinical condition should be achievable. A full functional assessment, treatment of any exacerbating physical or psychiatric disorder, and the provision of day care or assistance at home will be beneficial.
- However, dementia is a chronic progressive condition. The likely pattern may depend on the underlying pathology.

CASE 5.2 – **Behavioural problems in dementia**

A1: What is the likely differential diagnosis?

Preferred diagnosis:
- Deterioration in progressive dementia.

Alternative diagnoses:
- Delirium superimposed on dementia.
- Comorbid psychiatric diagnosis such as depression.

A2: What information in the history supports the diagnosis, and what other information would help to confirm it?

- It may be that his dementia is becoming worse. In the late stages of dementia increasing confusion, perceptual symptoms and memory loss may lead to aggression. The history may suggest Lewy body dementia. This is a dementia characterized by confusion, fluctuating cognitive deficits, psychotic symptoms, falls and mild extrapyramidal features. This may be difficult to distinguish from delirium. Lewy bodies are the pathological hallmark of Parkinson's disease – hence the extrapyramidal features. Such patients are also particularly prone to extrapyramidal side effects, so treatment with antipsychotic medication must be carried out with great caution.
- Delirium is common and coexists with dementia. It can exacerbate the symptoms of dementia. Screen for infection, drugs and metabolic abnormalities.
- The features that suggest Lewy body dementia (fluctuating clinical picture, confusion, perceptual symptoms) also occur in delirium.
- A depressive episode may lead to a reversible deterioration in cognitive function, as well as increased irritability, aggression or other behavioural disturbance.
- You need to take a full history from the wife and – as far as possible – also from the patient, looking for the symptoms and signs that may suggest one or other of your differential diagnoses. You would also need to check his prescribed medication and perform a physical examination to look for signs of physical illness that may be causing a reversible deterioration. You need to carefully ask the wife about the current level of social support being provided and find out how she is coping – carer mental illness is common in such situations, and the possibility of carer abuse should always be borne in mind. Ask specifically about dangerous behaviours, such as wandering and leaving things on the hob, and quantify his level of aggression and risk to his wife.

A3: What might the important aetiological factors be?

PREDISPOSING FACTORS

Predisposing factors for dementia include a family history of Alzheimer's disease, cardiovascular problems or diabetes. The patient's premorbid personality may be relevant to their current aggressive behaviour.

PRECIPITATING FACTORS

Social stressors or physical illness may lead to a clinical deterioration.

MAINTAINING FACTORS

Ongoing stresses or illness.

A4: What treatment options are available?

LOCATION

- This patient requires admission to hospital. It would not be possible to investigate him adequately as an outpatient, he is engaging in potentially dangerous behaviours, and his wife needs a rest.
- His capacity to agree to treatment must be assessed. It may be necessary to assess him for admission under the Mental Capacity Act or the Mental Health Act (MHA).

PHYSICAL

- The first step in management is identifying and treating any reversible causes of his delirium.
- Constipation, systemic infection, electrolyte imbalances and polypharmacy can all be corrected.
- Visual or hearing impairment can be addressed.
- Psychotic symptoms in dementia may be treated with antipsychotic medication. However, organic brain disease predicts a poor response.

PSYCHOLOGICAL

- Reassurance, problem-solving and support are as important in the elderly as in younger adults.
- Orientation therapy aims to provide repetitive reminders and cues orientating the patient to their current location and the current time.

SOCIAL

- Once his condition has been improved as much as possible, you need to consider further placement.
- Occupational therapy staff can carry out assessment of daily functioning in hospital and at home.
- His wife should be involved in the development of his care plan.
- In general, patients should be supported in their own home. Regular periods of respite care in hospital may help a carer to cope. Otherwise, residential or nursing home placement should be considered.

A5: What is the prognosis in this case?

Treatment of comorbid psychiatric or physical illness, management of functional deficits and support for his carers will lead to an improvement in his clinical condition. However, his dementia will continue to progress and the outlook in patients with dementia and behavioural problems is poor.

CASE 5.3 – **Persecutory ideas developing in old age**

A1: What is the likely differential diagnosis?

Preferred diagnosis:

- Late-onset schizophrenia (sometimes known as paraphrenia).

Alternative diagnoses:

- Dementia with organic psychotic symptoms.
- Depressive episode with psychotic symptoms.

A2: What information in the history supports the diagnosis, and what other information would help to confirm it?

- Paraphrenia is a non-affective psychosis of late onset that presents with similar symptoms to paranoid schizophrenia. It is considered to be a mild variant of schizophrenia. It is not characterized by prominent negative symptoms or personality deterioration. The presentation described is typical of this illness.
- To confirm the diagnosis you would try to demonstrate the presence of symptoms characteristic of schizophrenia. Therefore, you would confirm that her persecutory thoughts are indeed delusional, and then look for other symptoms of schizophrenia such as third-person auditory hallucinations or passivity phenomena.
- There are no specific indicators of cognitive decline. However, some of her beliefs might be due to poor short-term memory (e.g. forgetting where she has put things), and psychotic symptoms like these are common in dementia. You would need to exclude dementia, initially by using a screening test such as the MMSE.
- There are no specific features suggestive of depression, but this is a common illness and must be excluded.

A3: What might the important aetiological factors be?

PREDISPOSING FACTORS

People with paranoid or sensitive premorbid personalities are more likely to develop paraphrenia. It is also more common in people who are socially isolated, including those who have impaired hearing or vision.

PRECIPITATING FACTORS

It is common for illnesses such as this to present after the death of a supportive partner.

MAINTAINING FACTORS

Ongoing social isolation, life stresses and personality factors all may maintain the illness.

A4: What treatment options are available?

LOCATION

- This will take into account the severity and intrusiveness of her symptoms, consideration of any risk that may be posed to herself (self-harm and self-neglect) and others, the level of support she has at home from family and carers and the need for any further physical investigation or treatment.
- Given that she lives alone and has distressing psychotic symptoms, hospital admission may well be desirable.
- Attempts to achieve this voluntarily should be made, but if necessary the MHA may be used.

PHYSICAL

Paraphrenia is a non-affective psychosis, and is treated with antipsychotic medication. Those drugs with strong anticholinergic side effects or those that cause postural hypotension should be avoided in the elderly.

PSYCHOLOGICAL

Support, reassurance and explanation of symptoms are important. Ensuring that her hearing aid is appropriate and operational may help to reduce isolation and misinterpretations.

SOCIAL

- Day hospital or day centre attendance may reduce her isolation and improve her social network.
- Other problems such as financial help or provision of physical aids to mobility or independence in the home may improve her quality of life and reduce stress, thereby reducing the risk of relapse/recurrence.

A5: What is the prognosis in this case?

- The psychosis usually responds to antipsychotic treatment.
- Good prognostic factors include a quick response to treatment, younger age, and being married.
- If the disorder is long-standing, the prognosis is poor and the symptoms are likely to persist.

CASE 5.4 – **Severe low mood in old age**

A1: What is the likely differential diagnosis?

Preferred diagnosis:

- Severe depressive episode.

Alternative diagnoses:

- Generalized anxiety disorder.
- Delirium, possibly in the setting of underlying dementia.

A2: What information in the history supports the diagnosis, and what other information would help to confirm it?

- In older people depressive episodes are often characterized by psychomotor symptoms, that is, retarded depression or agitated depression. Psychotic symptoms are also more common. This case sounds very typical of agitated depression in which anxiety is typically a prominent symptom.
- A full history and MSE should reveal a depressive syndrome. You need to ask this woman about her mood and thoughts, looking for low mood and negative thoughts of hopelessness and helplessness, impending doom, poverty, illness and imminent death. In addition, she may describe biological symptoms of depression. She may have psychotic symptoms, almost certainly relating to her depression, such as nihilistic or hypochondriacal delusions or insulting auditory hallucinations (usually in the second person).
- Because of her apparent anxiety, you might consider an anxiety disorder as a diagnosis if there were no further symptoms of depression, but depression is more likely because of the acute onset of severe symptoms.
- Delirium may be suggested by the florid presentation and the acute onset. Delirium occurs very commonly in older people with many causes, particularly prescribed drugs (e.g. anticholinergics), metabolic disturbances, infection (urinary tract infection, chest infection) and constipation. It is particularly likely to occur in a patient who has a dementia. A simple cognitive screen and the exclusion of the characteristic symptoms of delirium should rule out this diagnosis.

A3: What might the important aetiological factors be?

PREDISPOSING FACTORS

A personal or family history of depression and an abnormal premorbid personality may be important.

PRECIPITATING FACTORS

Although this woman previously seemed independent, she may in fact have relied on her son's proximity. His holiday may have precipitated the episode.

MAINTAINING FACTORS

Ongoing social isolation, life stresses and personality factors may maintain the illness.

A4: What treatment options are available?

LOCATION

This woman needs to be admitted to hospital. She is elderly, lives alone, is severely unwell and distressed. Her self care and care of her home has been deteriorating. In addition, she will need investigation to exclude any underlying dementia or physical illness that may be contributing to the presentation.

PHYSICAL

- Depression in older people is treated in a similar way to depression in younger adults. It is necessary to consider the side effect profile of the antidepressant and to choose one without strong anticholinergic effects (which may precipitate confusion) or a strong hypotensive effect.
- If psychotic symptoms are present, combination treatment with an antipsychotic is necessary.

- Electroconvulsive therapy (ECT) is particularly effective in older people. Response of depression to ECT is predicted by the presence of psychotic symptoms, psychomotor symptoms and biological symptoms of depression. Therefore, in this case you would be likely to consider ECT early.

PSYCHOLOGICAL

- Initially, reassurance, explanation and development of a therapeutic relationship are necessary.
- Cognitive therapy is an effective treatment for depression. However, she is currently too severely ill to be able to benefit from this. It may be helpful as she recovers.

SOCIAL

Once she is recovering, you may need to further evaluate her day-to-day functioning and her level of support at home, and consider the need for further social support after discharge.

A5: What is the prognosis in this case?

- You would expect an acute depressive episode such as this to respond well to treatment.
- However, depression tends to recur. Continuation and maintenance antidepressant treatment reduce the likelihood of relapse and recurrence.

👫 OSCE counselling cases

OSCE COUNSELLING CASE 5.1

You have recently diagnosed an elderly widower as having dementia. Although his cognitive function is quite severely impaired, he has expressed a wish to remain at home and you have decided to support him in this for now. His daughter asks to see you because she is very concerned about his ability to live independently. She thinks that he needs to be placed in a home.

A1: What issues would you discuss with her?

- Listen carefully to the daughter's concerns. It is important to give relatives time to clearly explain their concerns, and enable you to develop a good relationship with them.
- Explain what assessments you have made, and the importance of her father's opinion.
- Explain what measures you have taken to enable him to live safely.
- Explain the prognosis, and what further measures will be available.
- Reassure her that assessment and monitoring will be ongoing, that she will be involved, that her opinion is important, and that if his situation at home becomes untenable, then residential care will be available.

REVISION PANEL

- A social assessment is especially important when dealing with elderly patients, to take account of issues related to bereavement, changes in social identity and roles, as well as their needs related to independent living skills.
- Always think about physical illness in elderly patients. It is common for physical illness to precipitate and maintain changes in mental state or behaviour, especially in the presence of an underlying dementia.
- You must include carers in your assessments, both in order to gain a complete picture of the patient, and also to consider whether the carer has mental health problems which may be contributing to your patient's presentation.
- Pharmacological treatment should be used cautiously in the elderly, often using lower doses than in younger adults. Polypharmacy is a common cause of mental and physical ill-health.

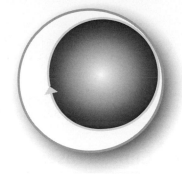

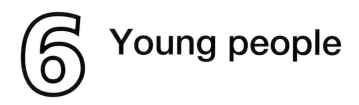

6 Young people

Questions

Clinical cases

For each of the case scenarios given, consider the following:

> **Q1**: What is the likely differential diagnosis?
> **Q2**: What information in the history supports the diagnosis, and what other information would help to confirm it?
> **Q3**: What might the important aetiological factors be?
> **Q4**: What treatment options are available?
> **Q5**: What is the prognosis in this case?

CASE 6.1 – **Failure to attend school**

An 11-year-old girl has been referred by her general practitioner (GP) because she has not been going to school. She has been complaining of abdominal pain, nausea and headaches. The GP has not found any underlying cause for her symptoms, and she has not had any weight loss. She is the youngest of four children, and has always been very conscientious and does well at school. Her mother has recently been in hospital for an operation.

On assessment, all of the family members seem anxious. The girl is quite tearful, but cheers up as the interview progresses and makes good eye contact. She says that she enjoys school when she gets there, but has found the move up to secondary school difficult and she does not like leaving her mother.

CASE 6.2 – **Behavioural problems in the classroom**

An 8-year-old boy is repeatedly in trouble at school. He has been threatened with suspension after he was verbally and physically aggressive to his teacher. The school have suggested that he has a problem with his concentration and advised his parents to ask the GP to refer him to child psychiatry. You see the boy with his parents and his younger sister. Unlike his sister, he keeps wriggling in his seat. His mother says his concentration is fine when he is playing on his computer. What worries her is that he does not seem to think before he does things and will run out across the road without looking.

CASE 6.3 – **Strange behaviour**

An 8-year-old boy has been referred because both his teachers and parents are concerned by what they describe as his 'strange behaviour'. He has always been a solitary child and does not have many friends. He likes to collect pebbles that he arranges in lines in his bedroom. He barks and makes high-pitched squeaks for no apparent reason. What bothers his parents most is that he will have tantrums for no obvious reason and he does not respond to being punished or rewarded. He is in mainstream school and seems to enjoy it, although he is 'often in a world of his own'. He loves copying cartoon characters in great detail.

At assessment he makes no eye contact with you, but tells you all about his pebble collection. His grammar and vocabulary seem normal, but his speech is stilted and he does not seem to realize that you are losing interest in what he is saying.

CASE 6.4 – **Faecal soiling**

A 9-year-old boy has been referred for constipation and faecal soiling. The GP has been using a combination of lactulose and senna for over a year, without much improvement. The boy is now refusing to do physical education (PE) at school, and his mother is annoyed that she still has to clean his soiled clothes.

When you meet them, he is very embarrassed. He passes large hard stools on an irregular basis, and semi-liquid faeces in between. His parents separated when he was 3 years old, and his mother thinks that this, combined with her depression, have caused the problems. She feels guilty, incompetent and angry.

CASE 6.5 – **Behavioural problems in a child with learning disabilities**

A 15-year-old boy with moderate mental retardation and autistic features is referred to you. He is able to speak, and can understand simple sentences. You are asked to see him at home because he has become increasingly agitated and is not communicating with anyone. According to his parents he is normally a happy boy, but over the past few weeks has become more withdrawn and quiet. The only recent change in his environment is that his daytime carer has been replaced. He is sitting on his bed and staring at the wall. He is mumbling to himself and appears to be responding to something that you cannot hear or see.

CASE 6.6 – **Low weight and low mood in a young girl**

A 14-year-old girl has been brought to the outpatient department by her mother who is very worried about how thin she has become over the past 6 months. The girl has been withdrawn and unhappy since her parents separated, and the GP is concerned that she may be depressed. At interview she makes little eye contact and insists there is nothing wrong. She does not think she is too thin and would like to lose more weight. It is difficult to see how thin she is because she is wearing layers of baggy clothes. She has not yet started her periods.

On examination, she has cold peripheries and her skin is dry. Her blood pressure is 110/60 mmHg, with no postural drop, and she is bradycardic. Her body weight is less than 85 per cent of her expected weight according to her age and height.

♟ OSCE counselling cases

OSCE COUNSELLING CASE 6.1

A 15-year-old girl is referred to you because her mother says she cannot care for her anymore. Over the past year the girl has been shoplifting, smoking and getting drunk regularly, and recently she has started cutting her arms. On assessment you are concerned by the girl's behaviour and the relationship between the girl and her mother. Your main concern is that her mother seems to be depressed.

Q1: How would you address this?

🔑 Key concepts

There are a number of important differences between child and adult mental disorders, both in their expression and in their management.

- Children live within, and are dependent on, their families. They are usually brought to medical attention by their parents who are concerned about some aspect of their development or behaviour. Their presentation is therefore dependent on the tolerance and expectations of the adults around them. Problems within children's families (e.g. parental mental illness or divorce) may affect them detrimentally. Other factors may also be protective (e.g. a supportive and stable relationship with one adult such as a grandparent). It is therefore essential that the clinician makes an assessment of the child's family and parents. A child's behaviour may be seen as an expression of distress within the family rather than solely to do with the child.
- Children are developing, and what is normal at one stage may not be at another. It is considered normal for a 3-year-old to wet the bed at night, but not a 10-year-old. Environmental events will have a different impact, depending on the age at which they occur. Separation from a parent is much harder for a toddler to cope with than an adolescent. Disorders may also present differently depending on the developmental stage of the child. Depressed children are often irritable, whereas depressed adolescents are able to describe feeling unhappy. Part of a child's assessment must therefore involve a developmental assessment.
- Children are less able than adults to express in words how they feel, and why they behave in the way they do. The clinician is thus more dependent on observing the child's behaviour and on reports from informants. Research has shown that informant reports have only a moderate agreement. This is partly due to children behaving differently in different environments, and also due to adults having different expectations and abilities to cope. This is another reason why a thorough exploration of a child's family and school experience is needed.
- As a result of all these complexities, child and adolescent psychiatrists take a systemic approach. The psychiatrist works as part of a multidisciplinary team that:
  - treats the child individually;
  - works with the whole family;
  - coordinates the efforts of all agencies involved with the child.

A SIMPLE OVERVIEW OF CHILD PSYCHIATRIC DISORDERS

Children can experience a number of the symptoms and disorders covered in the adult sections of this book, such as anxiety, depression and psychoses. The way these problems present will differ depending on the child's developmental stage. There are also some disorders that usually start during childhood or only occur in childhood. These fall into the following groups, which are based on the International Classification of Diseases (ICD)-10 classification:

1. Specific developmental disorders, e.g. specific reading disorder.
2. Pervasive developmental disorders, e.g. autism.
3. Hyperkinetic disorders.
4. Conduct disorders.
5. Emotional disorders, e.g. separation anxiety disorder.
6. Disorders of social functioning, e.g. attachment disorders or elective mutism.
7. Tic disorders, e.g. Gilles de la Tourette syndrome.
8. Other symptomatic disorders with onset during childhood, e.g. non-organic enuresis and encopresis.

Answers

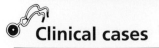

Clinical cases

CASE 6.1 – **Failure to attend school**

A1: What is the likely differential diagnosis?

Preferred diagnosis:

- Separation anxiety.

Alternative diagnoses:

- No underlying psychiatric problem.
- Physical health problem.
- Specific phobia.
- Depression.
- Psychosis.

A2: What information in the history supports the diagnosis, and what other information would help to confirm it?

- This is school refusal rather than truanting, because the girl's parents are aware that she is not going to school. In many cases of school refusal there is no underlying psychiatric diagnosis, but a child's anxiety, combined with their parents' inability or unwillingness to enforce attendance, lead to the child not going to school.
- Separation anxiety is suggested because she does not like leaving her mother. A careful developmental history should explore:
  - how she has coped with separation in the past;
  - her relationship with her mother and other members of the family;
  - any thoughts or fears she may have in relation to her mother's recent operation;
  - the timing of the physical symptoms. If they occur on a Sunday night, but not on a Friday night, this would point towards them being expressions of anxiety about school.
- She enjoys school when she gets there, and does well. This makes it unlikely to be a school-based problem. The school should be contacted (with parental consent) for information about her progress both academically and socially. Is the school aware of any problems (e.g. bullying)?
- Sometimes parents may withhold children from school, and this can be difficult to differentiate from school refusal when the parents are anxious and collude with the child.
- The GP has found no physical cause for her symptoms, so it is likely that these are somatic expressions of anxiety.
- It is important to ask about how she copes with leaving her mother for other reasons (e.g. going to a party). This will help to differentiate between separation anxiety and a specific phobia involving school.
- The girl cheers up during the interview and makes good eye contact. She describes enjoying school. This makes a diagnosis of depression unlikely.
- Psychosis, while rare, should always be considered.

A3: What might the important aetiological factors be?

PREDISPOSING FACTORS

- Poor parental discipline.
- Youngest children are probably at greater risk.
- Emotional over-involvement with the child.

PRECIPITATING FACTORS

Moving to a new school or a break from school due to holidays or illness.

MAINTAINING FACTORS

Parental collusion.

A4: What treatment options are available?

LOCATION

Treatment is usually as an outpatient.

PHYSICAL

There is no specific pharmacological treatment for school refusal, though medication may be considered if there is an underlying mental illness such as a depressive episode or psychosis.

PSYCHOLOGICAL

- It important for the whole family to make explicit the pattern of the symptoms and understand why they are occurring.
- If the child has had somatic symptoms, then the family needs to be reassured that there is no physical problem and to understand how anxiety can cause something like stomach ache.
- The parents need to be convinced of the importance of getting the child back to school, not only for their academic progress but also for their social development and self-confidence.
- Family therapy can help the parents lay down consistent rules that are carried through. It may also help to reduce emotional over-involvement.
- If the child has only been absent for a short time then a rapid return to school may be most effective. If the absence is more long term, a gradual desensitization approach may be more effective.

SOCIAL

Close liaison with the school and education welfare officers.

A5: What is the prognosis in this case?

- The majority of children successfully return to school and have no further problems.
- Younger children who have not been off school for long and receive help quickly have the best prognosis. There is an increased risk of school refusal in the future.
- Most children will go on to have no further problems in adulthood, but there is an increased risk of anxiety disorders and social problems.

CASE 6.2 – **Behavioural problems in the classroom**

A1: What is the likely differential diagnosis?

Preferred diagnosis:

- Hyperkinetic disorder.

Alternative diagnoses:

- Oppositional defiant disorder or conduct disorder.
- Emotional disorder (anxiety, depression or mania).
- Pervasive developmental disorder.
- Learning disability.
- Normality.

A2: What information in the history supports the diagnosis, and what other information would help to confirm it?

- His teachers think that he has a problem with concentration. The fact that he can concentrate on his computer is not contradictory, as many children with hyperkinetic disorder can concentrate on the television and on computer games where little active attention is required. In addition, he presents as overactive and his mother described impulsivity.
- The developmental history should demonstrate marked restlessness and inattentiveness that has persisted for at least 6 months and begun before 7 years of age. Ratings scales are commonly used to obtain information from parents and teachers (e.g. Conners' scales). This will help to establish that his symptoms occur both at school and at home. A school visit to observe him in class may be helpful as well as an educational psychology assessment.
- He has been in trouble at school. This may be as a result of his hyperactivity, poor concentration and impulsivity, but it may also be due to a conduct disorder. Both disorders involve impulsivity, and children with hyperkinetic disorder may also have a conduct disorder.
- A psychometric assessment should exclude learning difficulties. Children who do not understand or are bored may be inattentive and hyperactive.
- The history and mental state examination should exclude the other differential diagnoses.

A3: What might the important aetiological factors be?

PREDISPOSING FACTORS

There is a genetic contribution to hyperkinetic disorder, which is more common in boys than girls, and is more common in association with:

- Epilepsy.
- Learning disabilities.
- A history of perinatal obstetric complications.
- Prematurity.
- Maternal stress during pregnancy.
- Fetal exposure to alcohol, drugs and cigarettes.
- Low socioeconomic status or social deprivation.

PRECIPITATING FACTORS

Ongoing social stressors, such as poor family relationships, poor discipline at home or inconsistent parenting may precipitate a deterioration and presentation.

MAINTAINING FACTORS

Precipitating factors are likely to be ongoing and maintain the disorder.

A4: What treatment options are available?

LOCATION

Treatment should be as an outpatient.

PHYSICAL

- Methylphenidate is the most commonly used medication:
  - it improves attention and activity and so often results in improved ability to learn and get on with peers and family;
  - before commencing methylphenidate a neurological examination must be completed and height, weight and blood pressure measured;
  - side effects include appetite suppression and difficulty getting to sleep. The child may also become unhappy and tearful or develop tics or stereotypical movements;
  - the drug is usually well tolerated, and long-term use is safe. While on the drug the child must be followed up by a specialist;
  - there are a number of modified release forms of methylphenidate which can be used so the child only needs to take one pill in the morning.
- Exclusion diet. These have been found to be beneficial, but they are very difficult for families to maintain. There is no way of predicting which foodstuffs are responsible in any particular child.

PSYCHOLOGICAL

- Explaining the condition to the child, family and school is enormously helpful. When it is understood that the child is not behaving in this way on purpose, the pattern of the child being blamed all the time can be broken.
- Cognitive and behavioural approaches. The child needs rapid rewards when they manage to stay on task. Rules about unacceptable behaviour must be clear and sanctions consistent. Parent training classes and teacher training can create consistency for the child.

SOCIAL

Close liaison with the school and education welfare officers is important.

A5: What is the prognosis in this case?

- Symptoms usually decrease during adolescence, although some people continue to be hyperactive and have difficulties concentrating in adulthood.
- Children with hyperkinetic disorder and conduct disorder are at increased risk of substance misuse and antisocial personality disorder.

CASE 6.3 – **Strange behaviour**

A1: What is the likely differential diagnosis?

Preferred diagnosis:

- Asperger's syndrome.

Alternative diagnoses:

- Autism.
- Gilles de la Tourette syndrome.
- Obsessive–compulsive disorder.
- Learning disability.
- Degenerative disorder.

A2: What information in the history supports the diagnosis, and what other information would help to confirm it?

- He does not have any friends, and at interview he does not make eye contact and does not check to see whether you are interested in what he is saying. He is displaying features of impaired reciprocal social interaction. He has a preoccupation with pebbles and lining them up. This is suggestive of an autistic spectrum disorder.

- He is still in mainstream school, and his vocabulary and grammar seem normal. This makes it likely that his language development has not been seriously delayed (as occurs in autism). His speech is, however, qualitatively different. He does not grasp the normal give and take of conversation, and his speech is stilted with abnormal intonation (prosody). This is characteristic of Asperger's syndrome.
- Children with Asperger's syndrome often do not understand rules and find changes difficult, making rewards and punishments meaningless unless they are very simple. Chris may have tantrums as a result of changes in his routines that are so small that his parents do not notice them.
- A developmental history may demonstrate an initial period of normal development, but most children will have shown early signs of abnormal social interest or communication, e.g. not liking cuddles, not reaching to be picked up, or not pointing.
- It would be important to obtain information about his social skills, imagination and repetitive behaviour. In obsessive–compulsive disorder the compulsive behaviour is associated with anxiety; however, in autistic spectrum disorders the repetitive behaviour is reassuring and can be seen as a way in which the individual tries to structure a world which otherwise seems very confusing.
- Other investigations worth considering are:
  - Psychometric assessment. Children with learning disabilities may have features of autistic disorder, and many children with autism are also learning disabled.
  - A communication and language assessment.
  - Information from his school (with parental consent) about his academic and social abilities.
  - A full physical examination to detect recognizable syndromes, particularly tuberous sclerosis, and any localizing neurological signs. This should also include hearing and visual acuity assessment.
  - Genetic testing for fragile X syndrome.

A3: What might the important aetiological factors be?

PREDISPOSING FACTORS

- Genetic: twin studies indicate a heritability of over 90 per cent, probably due to an adverse combination of a number of genes.
- A minority of cases of autism are associated with medical conditions such as tuberous sclerosis and fragile X syndrome.
- There has been debate about whether the measles, mumps and rubella vaccine (MMR) given at 1 year is associated with autism. The majority opinion is that there is no good evidence of a link.

PRECIPITATING FACTORS

Severe and prolonged early deprivation may result in autistic symptoms, but there is no evidence that early traumatic events or poor parenting actually cause autism.

MAINTAINING FACTORS

Social stressors such as family discord or difficulties in peer relationships, life events or any changes in routine or environment may lead to a worsening of his symptoms.

A4: What treatment options are available?

LOCATION

Treatment should be as an outpatient.

PHYSICAL

- There are no specific pharmacological treatments for autistic spectrum disorders.
- Associated problems such as seizures, hyperactivity, aggression or anxiety should be treated as appropriate.

PSYCHOLOGICAL

- Making a diagnosis, explaining the child's difficulties and behaviour and providing support to the parents can in itself be enormously helpful to the family and child.
- Children with autistic spectrum disorders respond best in structured environments with consistent behavioural programmes both at school and home.

SOCIAL

- The National Autistic Society can be very supportive to families.
- Appropriate school placement. Some children with Asperger's syndrome manage in mainstream school especially if there is an autistic unit attached to it.
- Liaison with social services and education.

A5: What is the prognosis in this case?

- The best predictors of outcome are non-verbal IQ and linguistic ability. Children with higher IQs and fluent speech at 5 years of age are more likely to achieve independent living, but most do not marry or become parents.
- Much depends on the support of an individual's family and their local services in setting up an environment in which the person can cope.
- There is an increased risk of seizures in adolescence.

CASE 6.4 – **Faecal soiling**

A1: What is the likely differential diagnosis?

Preferred diagnosis:

- Encopresis due to constipation with overflow.

Alternative diagnoses:

- Failure to toilet train.
- A specific phobia.
- Stressful experiences.

A2: What information in the history supports the diagnosis, and what other information would help to confirm it?

- Encopresis is a term that is used to describe any sort of inappropriate deposition of faeces (including in the pants after 4 years of age). It is sometimes used specifically to refer to the deposition of normal stools in inappropriate places, such as in a drawer or the freezer.
- The history suggests that this boy has constipation with large faecal plugs developing in his rectum. This results in further retention and a stretching of the rectum and an associated loss of sensation. Semi-liquid faeces may be leaking around the blockage. His parents' separation at the time he was toilet training may have resulted in him not acquiring normal bowel control. His mother's depression may have contributed to this further, or may have resulted in a stress-induced loss of bowel control.
- A thorough developmental history focusing particularly on toilet training is required. This should determine whether he has ever been faecally continent, and whether there was an initial cause for his constipation (low-fibre diet, anal fissure, deliberate retention). Enquiries should be made about delays in any other areas (e.g. enuresis).
- A detailed history of the problem must find out whether anything has made it better or worse, how the different family members respond to it, and which treatment strategies have been used. In addition, an assessment of his diet would be useful. The mother should be asked if he has ever been provocative with his soiling (e.g. passed stool on furniture or smeared his faeces).
- His anxieties about toileting need to be explored to exclude a specific phobia.

- Other useful investigations would include:
  - an assessment of the family dynamics;
  - a physical examination;
  - a school report (with parental consent) of academic and social progress.

A3: What might the important aetiological factors be?

PREDISPOSING FACTORS

Only family studies have been done, but these do suggest a genetic contribution.

PRECIPITATING FACTORS

- It has been suggested that earlier toilet training and family factors such as lack of parental sensitivity, family disorganization or a reluctance to foster independence in the child may result in problems in toilet training and faecal incontinence.
- Sexual abuse can be associated with constipation and soiling.
- Stresses both within the family and outside it may lead to constipation and soiling as a result of anxiety or anger.

MAINTAINING FACTORS

The boy's embarrassment and his mother's frustration and anger may be maintaining the problem.

A4: What treatment options are available?

LOCATION

Treatment will almost always be as an outpatient. A liaison approach with paediatricians is most appropriate.

PHYSICAL

Evacuation of the bowel followed by the use of laxatives to prevent stool from reaccumulating. A regular bowel habit is then encouraged.

PSYCHOLOGICAL

- Explanation to the parents and child of the pathophysiology of the problem can help to reduce embarrassment and anger and enable the parents and child to work together to address the problem.
- A cognitive behavioural approach using positive reinforcement (operant conditioning) with a star chart and associated rewards is used.
- A family therapy approach has also been used in which the problem is externalized and the therapist and child fight against the 'sneaky poo'.

SOCIAL

As with all child cases, it is important to fully involve the family in the management.

A5: What is the prognosis in this case?

It is very rare for soiling to persist into adulthood. Chronic courses are more likely where the soiling is associated with other problems such as family difficulties, other psychiatric disorders or school problems.

CASE 6.5 – **Behavioural problems in a child with learning disabilities**

A1: What is the likely differential diagnosis?

Preferred diagnosis:

- Acute psychotic episode.

Alternative diagnoses:

- Physical illness (urinary tract infection, chest infection, complex partial status epilepticus).
- A reaction to stress (e.g. change in routine or carers, some form of abuse).
- Affective disorder.
- Side effects of medication.

A2: What information in the history supports the diagnosis, and what other information would help to confirm it?

- Assessing people with learning disabilities can be difficult if their language development is limited, making diagnosis dependent on informant histories from people who know the person well. A full history from all those involved in his care is needed.
- Mental illness is much more common in people with learning disabilities, but it may not follow the same patterns as an individual's experiences or feelings may be communicated and expressed in a different way.
- He has been increasingly quiet and withdrawn over the past few weeks. He now appears to be responding to hallucinations. This may suggest that he has schizophrenia. Alternatively, depression may cause social withdrawal and psychotic symptoms.
- A full medical history and physical examination (including vision and hearing assessment) is essential. People with learning disabilities have increased rates of epilepsy and other neurological disabilities. They are also more likely to have physical disability and associated physical illness including delirium. Side effects from medication may not follow normal patterns, and should be considered carefully.
- One of his carers has recently been replaced. This may have distressed him enormously. Other possible stressors must also be considered. People with learning disabilities are vulnerable to abuse, and they also experience more stigma and social isolation than people who are not learning-disabled.
- It is important to consider his risk of harm to himself or to others, or whether he is at risk of self-neglect.

A3: What might the important aetiological factors be?

PREDISPOSING FACTORS

These may include poor communication skills, increased experience of failure leading to low expectations of success and global negative self-evaluation, impaired social understanding, increased vulnerability to abuse, social stigma or neurodevelopmental lesions of the medial temporal lobe.

PRECIPITATING FACTORS

Possibilities include seizures or other neurological abnormalities associated with the learning disability, subacute delirium, medication side effects, illicit drug use, family stress and lack of peer support.

MAINTAINING FACTORS

Ongoing stressors or changes in environment.

A4: What treatment options are available?

LOCATION

A period of assessment as an inpatient may be appropriate, but this could cause him even more distress. This should be considered by the multidisciplinary team looking after him, as well as his parents.

PHYSICAL

- Antipsychotic medication would treat his psychosis and agitation.
- Side effects such as sedation, acute dystonia, tardive dyskinesia and lowering of the seizure threshold need to be considered. Therefore, an atypical antipsychotic should be chosen.

PSYCHOLOGICAL

Support, reassurance and education about illness are as important in those with learning disabilities as those without. However, obviously this needs to be tailored to the abilities of each individual.

SOCIAL

Support of his family and other carers.

A5: What is the prognosis in this case?

- It is likely that he would respond to antipsychotic medication in the short term.
- He will be at risk of further episodes of psychosis, particularly at times of stress, and might develop negative symptoms of schizophrenia.
- The prognosis of schizophrenia may be worse in those with learning disabilities because they are likely to be more vulnerable to stress and have limited coping strategies.
- A psychiatric illness will place an even greater burden on his family, who may find it hard to cope.

CASE 6.6 – **Low weight and low mood in a young girl**

A1: What is the likely differential diagnosis?

Preferred diagnosis:

- Anorexia nervosa.

Alternative diagnoses:

- Depressive episode.
- Physical illness (e.g. gastrointestinal disease, chronic debilitating disease).
- Obsessive–compulsive disorder.

A2: What information in the history supports the diagnosis, and what other information would help to confirm it?

- This case has a number of features suggestive of anorexia nervosa. The girl's weight is less than 85 per cent of her expected weight according to her height and age, but despite this she does not consider herself to be thin (body image distortion). Her menarche is delayed. It is necessary to establish that her weight loss is self-induced, for example by avoiding fattening foods and/or by self-induced vomiting, purging, exercise or use of diuretics/appetite suppressants.
- It is common for patients with anorexia nervosa to complain of depressive symptoms. Depressive symptoms may be the result of semi-starvation, which can cause low mood, social isolation and insomnia. Sometimes depressive symptoms merit an additional diagnosis, but usually this can be reassessed once the person has gained some weight.
- Physical illness resulting in severe weight loss is not usually accompanied by a fear of fatness or body image distortion.

- A full history should explore the development of her symptoms and explore an understanding of her current life with respect to interpersonal relationships, her family, boyfriends, peers at school, etc. Assessment of her personality is also likely to be important.
- The physical signs of anorexia nervosa include:
  - lanugo hair;
  - hypertrophy of the parotid and salivary glands;
  - loss of or failure to develop secondary sexual characteristics;
  - pitting on the teeth due to enamel erosion, and calluses on the back of the hands (due to self-induced vomiting);
  - osteoporosis (decreased oestrogen and low calcium intake and absorption);
  - renal impairment (hypokalaemia and chronic dehydration);
  - normochromic normocytic anaemia;
  - cardiac arrhythmia.
- Initial investigations would include:
  - full blood count, urea and electrolytes, liver function tests, thyroid function tests, glucose;
  - baseline electrocardiogram;
  - ultrasound scanning of the ovaries – this may be useful to monitor disease progress.

A3: What might the important aetiological factors be?

PREDISPOSING FACTORS

- Twin and family studies suggest that there is a genetic contribution.
- A premorbid personality involving perfectionism and dependence.
- A poor body image.

PRECIPITATING FACTORS

Perceived encouragement to diet from family, peers and the media.

MAINTAINING FACTORS

The 'reward' of weight loss and the feeling of being 'in control'.

A4: What treatment options are available?

LOCATION

- Inpatient treatment should be considered if weight is less than 70 per cent of the expected weight, if the patient is physically compromised (bradycardia and postural hypotension), if there is very rapid weight loss, if depression is severe or there is a risk of self-harm, or if outpatient treatment has failed.
- The Mental Health Act may be used to admit a very ill person against their will.

PHYSICAL

Drugs have a limited role in treatment, though antidepressants may be useful, particularly in the presence of depressive symptoms.

PSYCHOLOGICAL

- The first goal is to increase weight gradually. This is usually achieved by eating an increased number of small meals. A dietician will help the young person to plan their intake and calculate the number of calories required. Weight and physical state need to be regularly monitored.
- A combination of family therapy, individual therapy and behavioural work is used as an outpatient service, unless the case is very severe. The family work aims to help the parents to take responsibility for the young person's weight gain and to work with any family difficulties. Weight gain is rewarded, and the individual work aims to educate the person about dieting, their illness and its effects.

Problem-solving techniques, cognitive behavioural work and support are also important. Research seems to show that patients over 18 years of age do better with an individual approach, whereas those who are 18 years or under benefit from a more family-orientated approach.

SOCIAL

It may be necessary to liaise with her school and social services about her ongoing care.

A5: What is the prognosis in this case?

- About 50 per cent of cases recover, 30 per cent are improved, and 20 per cent become chronic. A small number may develop bulimia nervosa. The mortality rate is less than 5 per cent.
- Good prognostic factors include early age of onset, a good parent–child relationship, and rapid detection and treatment.
- Poor prognostic factors include binge eating, vomiting, premorbid problems and chronicity.

⚹ OSCE counselling cases

OSCE COUNSELLING CASE 6.1

A 15-year-old girl is referred to you because her mother says she cannot care for her anymore. Over the past year the girl has been shoplifting, smoking and getting drunk regularly, and recently she has started cutting her arms. On assessment you are concerned by the girl's behaviour and the relationship between the girl and her mother. Your main concern is that her mother seems to be depressed.

A1: How would you address this?

- When a young person is brought as the patient with the problem it is very difficult to introduce the idea that other members of the family may have problems and be a part of the young person's difficulties. Engaging the family and developing a rapport is essential.
- Listen and empathize with the situations of both the mother and the daughter. This may also help to lessen the conflict between them.
- It may be helpful to see them individually. This will give them an opportunity to say things in private and perhaps to express difficulties more freely.
- If the mother does not describe any symptoms of depression you may need to gently suggest this to her. This may be a process that occurs over a number of sessions. When she is able to acknowledge her problems you could offer to contact her GP to alert them to your concerns.
- If you take a systemic view, then families are often quick to start making links too. For example, you might notice similarities in the ways that mother and daughter approach problems or express feelings. Drawing a family tree and making links with other generations can also help this view.
- Depending on the individuals and their relationship you may decide that a family therapy approach is most helpful, and/or individual work with the girl and her mother.
- If the girl and her mother agreed, it would be very important to work with any other members of the family, the girl's school, and any other agencies involved – for example, the youth offending team and social services.

REVISION PANEL

- Most children live in families and are dependent on the adults who care for them. This affects the way in which they present for help and the way in which they must be assessed.
- Children are on a developmental trajectory. Where they are in this process must be assessed so that you can judge where they should be, what is normal behaviour and what their needs are.
- Because children may be less able to express their difficulties, taking histories from other sources (parents, teachers, friends) is very important.
- The child psychiatrist works within a multidisciplinary team and must also be able to work effectively with the other agencies involved with a child (e.g. education, social care, criminal justice system).
- Children and young people experience many of the adult psychiatric disorders, but there are some disorders which are specific to childhood.

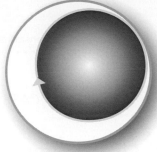

7 Psychiatry in general medical settings

Questions

Clinical cases

For each of the case scenarios given, consider the following:

> **Q1**: What is the likely differential diagnosis?
> **Q2**: What information in the history supports the diagnosis, and what other information would help to confirm it?
> **Q3**: What might the important aetiological factors be?
> **Q4**: What treatment options are available?
> **Q5**: What is the prognosis in this case?

CASE 7.1 – Overdose and self-cutting in a young woman

A 19-year-old woman presents to the accident and emergency department saying that she has taken an unknown number of sleeping tablets. In addition, she has a number of lacerations to her left forearm which appear to have been self-inflicted and which are bleeding profusely. She is accompanied by her boyfriend, who says that she took the pills and cut herself with a razor after they had had an argument. He immediately brought her to hospital. The general medical team has assessed her, dressed her wounds, and consider that she is physically fit to be discharged. The team tells you that she has presented in this way many times before and ask you to sanction her discharge.

CASE 7.2 – Mood disturbance, sleep disturbance and difficult behaviour in a general hospital

A 60-year-old man has been in hospital for a total of 5 days, having undergone a total hip replacement 3 days ago. He is becoming increasingly difficult to manage on the ward. He is argumentative with nursing staff, sleeping little at night, and disturbing other patients. His mood is changeable, being angry and hostile one minute and placid and calm the next. He has accused the nursing staff of being prison officers, preventing him from leaving.

CASE 7.3 – Physical symptoms with no demonstrable pathology

You are asked to see a woman on a general medical ward who has been an inpatient for 5 days undergoing investigation for pain in her loin. This was initially thought to be renal in origin, but an intravenous urethrogram was negative for stones and no other cause for her continued pain can be identified. In addition, it has been noted that she has presented to the hospital on a number of occasions over the past year or so complaining of a wide variety of symptoms and different pains for which no physical cause has been identified. The medical team has discussed these findings with the patient and told her that they want to get a psychiatric opinion.

CASE 7.4 – **Atypical seizures**

A 27-year-old woman was brought into hospital by her husband. She is said to have had epilepsy for some time. It is poorly controlled with a combination of anticonvulsants. Her husband says that she has had an increasing frequency of fits over the past 2 days. In view of the frequency of fits, she was admitted to hospital 3 days ago. She has continued to have up to four fits a day while an inpatient. The medical team is concerned that her seizures are atypical, and think they may not be due to epilepsy. They ask for a psychiatric opinion. Her husband is very concerned about her health, particularly as he is due to go abroad for 3 months soon to complete an important contract for work.

👫 OSCE counselling cases

OSCE COUNSELLING CASE 7.1

You are asked to see a patient in the accident and emergency department who has taken an overdose of paracetamol. He requires physical treatment for the effects of this in hospital, but is refusing.

Q1: What would you do and what advice would you give to the medical staff?

Q2: Explain how you would carry out an assessment of his risk of self-harm.

Key concepts

Psychiatric morbidity is common in general hospital and primary care settings, and is probably under-recognized. There is a variety of reasons for this:

- Both are common, and will often occur together by chance.
- Physical disorder may predispose to psychiatric disorder:
  - some physical disorders directly cause psychiatric symptoms or problems, such as delirium, endocrine disorders, drug toxicity, metabolic abnormalities, etc.;
  - physical disorders may indirectly cause psychiatric disorder. This is particularly likely in cases of chronic painful illness, illness which may endanger life or illness which requires unpleasant treatments.
- Psychiatric disorder may lead to physical disorders, for example alcohol dependence, eating disorders, deliberate self-harm.
- Psychiatric disorder may present with physical symptoms:
  - atypical depression, anxiety disorders, adjustment disorders, obsessive–compulsive disorder;
  - somatoform disorders – somatization disorder, hypochondriasis, persistent somatoform pain disorder.
- Each condition may affect the treatment response and prognosis of the other. It is important not to assume that psychological distress is merely a normal response to an unpleasant situation and unworthy of treatment. Individual patient factors are important in determining this relationship. Therefore, the liaison psychiatrist needs to pay particular attention to:
  - relevant personality traits or personality disorder;
  - personal and social stressors – occupation, marriage, finances, housing, other relationships, etc.

Treatment and management must be tailored to the patient. It is important to determine whether the patient is 'psychologically minded', or not. In other words, are they able to think about their problems in psychological terms? Clumsy attempts to discuss psychological causes for physical symptoms may lead to the patient feeling that their symptoms are being ignored, or that they are being accused of malingering. This requires great care and sensitivity.

Particular diagnoses that can cause confusion are the somatoform disorders and the dissociative (or conversion) disorders. Both groups of diagnoses share the idea that psychological distress may present with physical symptoms.

- In **somatoform disorders** (somatization disorder, hypochondriasis and persistent somatoform pain disorder) the complaint is of a physical symptom.
- In **dissociative disorders** on the other hand, there must in addition be some alteration in or loss of functioning.

A patient with persistent pain or persistent gastrointestinal symptoms may have a somatoform disorder, while the patient complaining of paralysis of a limb, or who presents with amnesia, has a dissociative disorder.

The assessment of capacity is often important in general medical settings. This was placed on a statutory footing for the first time by the Mental Capacity Act 2005.

- Mental capacity is 'decision specific and time specific'. This means that the question to ask is not 'Does this person have capacity?' but 'Can this person make this decision at this time?'
- Capacity is the ability to: understand the information pertinent to the decision; retain that information; weigh up the pros and cons of the decision; and communicate the decision made.

You should assume someone has capacity unless there is evidence to the contrary (this does not include an unusual or eccentric decision) and you should do all you can to maximize their capacity. If you are making a decision for someone who lacks capacity you must act in their best interests, choose the least restrictive option, consult their family and friends and consider their past and present views and beliefs. If the person is likely to regain capacity you should see if the decision can be delayed until they have improved sufficiently to make their own decision.

Answers

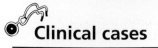 **Clinical cases**

CASE 7.1 – **Overdose and self-cutting in a young woman**

A1: What is the likely differential diagnosis?

Preferred diagnosis:

- Personality disorder, probably emotionally unstable.

Alternative diagnoses:

- Depression.
- No mental disorder.

A2: What information in the history supports the diagnosis, and what other information would help to confirm it?

- The history of repeated self-harm, which sounds impulsive as it occurred after an argument, is suggestive of personality disorder rather than acute mental illness. Impulsivity, which may lead to repeated self-harm, drug and alcohol misuse, criminal convictions and sexual promiscuity for example, is especially characteristic of emotionally unstable personality disorder. Such people also have instability of mood (often leading to episodes of low mood) and disturbed self-image (resulting in unclear goals and direction in life, perhaps ambivalence over sexual orientation). Patients may also complain of chronic feelings of emotional emptiness and a fear of abandonment. This type of personality disorder is strongly associated with a history of childhood sexual abuse.
- This diagnosis would be confirmed by taking a careful history, attempting to demonstrate the characteristic pattern of personality traits. These should be so extreme as to cause personal distress or significant problems in social functioning or interpersonal relationships. You also need to gather information from friends or relatives, and perhaps from other agencies such as social services.
- However, it is vital to exclude the presence of acute mental illness such as depression, which may be readily treatable and is more common in people with personality disorder.
- Alternatively, she may have no mental disorder, the self-harm being simply an impulsive gesture related to her relationship problems. However, her history of repetitive self-harm suggests otherwise.

A3: What might the important aetiological factors be?

PREDISPOSING FACTORS

Emotionally unstable personality disorder (which may be subdivided into impulsive and borderline types) is associated with a history of abuse in childhood. This may be physical, emotional or sexual abuse.

PRECIPITATING FACTORS

Her self-harm has been precipitated by an argument with her boyfriend.

MAINTAINING FACTORS

Personality disorders are chronic by nature.

A4: What treatment options are available?

LOCATION

- Generally, patients with this form of personality disorder do not do well as inpatients. The ward environment will reduce her ability to use her habitual coping mechanisms to deal with stress, and this may lead to increasing acting out and behavioural disturbance.
- However, inpatient treatment might be necessary either because she is at high risk of further self-harm in the short term, or because there is evidence that she is also suffering from a comorbid mental illness, probably a depressive episode.

PHYSICAL

- There is little place for medication in the treatment of emotionally unstable personality disorder.
- It has been suggested that low doses of depot antipsychotics may reduce suicidality, but the evidence is not conclusive.

PSYCHOLOGICAL

- This may take the form of a 'here and now' approach, aiming to support during crises and gradually helping the person to overcome their difficulties with for example, problem-solving therapy, cognitive therapies, anxiety management or assertiveness training.
- Alternatively, a psychodynamic approach could be taken. This would look at the patient's past life to try to identify problems in childhood that may have led to their current difficulties. Once identified, the patient is then encouraged to 'work through' these in therapy sessions. This is a long-term treatment which is dependent on the patient's ability to form a stable therapeutic relationship and their ability to withstand re-experiencing childhood trauma without self-harming or acting out in some other way. The impulsivity and other characteristics of emotionally unstable personality disorder often make this form of therapy unsuitable.
- Therapeutic communities provide a safe and stable environment in which a group of patients with such problems can live and work through their problems. However, this would not be suitable for a patient in an acute crisis. It might be an option when she has had a more settled period in the community.

SOCIAL

This will aim to reduce stresses and problems in the person's life which might precipitate episodes of mental illness or episodes of self-harm. Accommodation, financial or work-related issues are common causes of stress.

A5: What is the prognosis in this case?

- Personality disorders are defined as deeply ingrained, enduring abnormalities of mood and behaviour. Therefore, by definition they are chronic. However, they may improve somewhat with increasing age and it may be possible to ameliorate them and their negative impact on the patient with the treatment options described above.
- Rates of mental illness are raised among those with personality disorder, and the presence of personality disorder makes mental illness more difficult to treat.

CASE 7.2 – **Mood disturbance, sleep disturbance and difficult behaviour in a general hospital**

A1: What is the likely differential diagnosis?

Preferred diagnosis:

- Delirium.

Alternative diagnoses:

- Dementia.
- Delirium with underlying dementia.
- Mania.
- Schizophrenia or other psychosis.

A2: What information in the history supports the diagnosis, and what other information would help to confirm it?

- Delirium is suggested by his poor sleep at night and his rapidly changing mood. Information from nurses and relatives may be useful, particularly in relation to his condition prior to hospital admission, his medication history, and any history of alcohol misuse. Delirium would be confirmed by the presence of the other symptoms of the syndrome:
  - impaired attention and concentration, new learning, disorientation and disturbed consciousness;
  - muddled or rambling thought and speech, transient ideas of reference or delusions;
  - florid perceptual disturbance with visual illusions, misinterpretations and hallucinations, auditory hallucinations;
  - disturbed sleep–wake cycle – daytime sleepiness, poor sleep at night with worsening of symptoms;
  - rapid changes in mood state and psychomotor activity.
- The presentation is unlikely to be solely due to dementia because a dementia of this severity would almost certainly have been noted previously. However, delirium commonly complicates dementia. Features that would particularly distinguish delirium from dementia are:
  - gross disturbance of attention and concentration;
  - disorientation in time, place or person;
  - acute onset and fluctuating course.
- It is possible that this man's changing mood could be the lability of mood that is associated with mania, and his accusations of nursing staff could be the persecutory thoughts that may occur in psychosis. Features that would distinguish delirium from psychiatric causes of psychosis are:
  - florid visual hallucinations, illusions and misinterpretations;
  - no history of mental illness;
  - very rapidly changing picture with gross disturbance of cognitive function;
  - characteristic diurnal fluctuation in symptoms.

A3: What might the important aetiological factors be?

PREDISPOSING FACTORS

Delirium is more likely to occur in patients with previous brain disease, such as dementia.

PRECIPITATING FACTORS

- The delirium may be due to the anaesthetic, metabolic abnormalities, infection or other systemic or intracranial disease.
- Alcohol misuse is a common cause, through two main mechanisms:
  - delirium tremens (confusion, gross tremor and autonomic disturbance), due to acute alcohol withdrawal;
  - Wernicke's encephalopathy (confusion, ataxia and ophthalmoplegia), due to thiamine deficiency commonly secondary to alcohol dependence.

Physical investigations should help to determine the underlying cause (see Table 7.1)

Table 7.1 Investigations aiding in determining the cause of delirium

Investigation	Cause of delirium
Look at drug chart	Benzodiazepines, anticholinergics, narcotics
Full blood count, urea and electrolytes, liver function tests, blood glucose, calcium	Anaemia, infection, metabolic causes
Thyroid function tests	Hypothyroidism or hyperthyroidism
Electrocardiography	Cardiac failure
Temperature, pulse, chest radiograph, midstream urine	Infection
Computed tomography/magnetic resonance imaging of the head	If focal cerebral lesion
Electroencephalography	Generalized diffuse slowing may aid the diagnosis of delirium

MAINTAINING FACTORS

- These are the same as the precipitating factors.

A4: What treatment options are available?

LOCATION

- Delirium should be managed within a general hospital.

PHYSICAL

- The underlying cause must be identified and treated as appropriate.
- Medication should be avoided if possible because of its potential to exacerbate the delirium. However, occasionally it is necessary to mildly sedate a patient. There are two main options:
  - **antipsychotics** – haloperidol is usually preferred because of its relatively mild anticholinergic and cardiac effects. Small doses (0.5–10 mg/day) are usually effective, particularly in elderly patients. Atypical antipsychotics may also be effective, though at present there is less evidence relating to their use. Antipsychotics should be avoided in alcohol or sedative withdrawal because of the risk of seizures;
  - **benzodiazepines** may also be useful, particularly if side effects limit the use of antipsychotics, or in delirium due to alcohol or sedative withdrawal (they increase the seizure threshold). However, they may worsen cognitive impairment. Respiratory function and level of sedation need to be monitored closely.

PSYCHOLOGICAL

- Symptomatic treatment involves careful nursing.
- He should be kept in a quiet, well-lit side room with a dimmed light at night.
- Communication must be clear, simple and repetitive, orientating the patient to the time and day, location, identity of staff members.
- Any unnecessary objects, which may lead to misinterpretations, should be removed from the room.
- Staff should be as consistent as possible, with a minimum number of nurses caring for the patient.

A5: What is the prognosis in this case?

The prognosis of delirium is dependent on the underlying cause, but recovery is usual. There is an associated mortality, however, which is higher in delirium tremens because of the risk of seizures.

CASE 7.3 – **Physical symptoms with no demonstrable pathology**

A1: What is the likely differential diagnosis?

Preferred diagnosis:

- Somatization disorder.

Alternative diagnoses:

- Hypochondriasis.
- Atypical presentation of depression, anxiety disorder or adjustment disorder.
- Delusional disorder or other psychosis.
- Deliberate and conscious feigning of symptoms (malingering or factitious disorder).
- A physical pathology which has not been identified by investigations.

A2: What information in the history supports the diagnosis, and what other information would help to confirm it?

- In somatization disorder the patient has a preoccupation with the presence of various physical symptoms. The variability of her symptoms suggests that her preoccupation is with the symptoms themselves, rather than with having some serious underlying disease, as is the case in hypochondriasis. You need to carefully determine the nature of the woman's overvalued ideas about her symptoms to decide if somatization or hypochondriasis is the more appropriate diagnosis.
- A full history and mental state examination (MSE) will exclude an underlying psychiatric illness. You need to ask about the syndromes of depression and the anxiety disorders, and to see if there is any evidence of a recent stress which may have precipitated illness or an adjustment disorder.
- If her beliefs are delusional, then the diagnosis must be a psychosis – probably persistent delusional disorder in view of the duration of the symptoms.
- Malingering implies that there is a clear gain or reason for faking symptoms, such as to obtain opiates, to avoid work, or for financial compensation. In factitious disorder (or Munchausen's syndrome) on the other hand the reason is not clear, and is presumably related to the patient's personality or some internal psychopathology. Usually, these patients will discharge themselves when they are 'discovered', so if she remains in hospital after being told that no cause can be found, these diagnoses are relatively unlikely.
- Her repeated presentations to hospital with unexplained symptoms and repeated negative investigations suggest that there is no physical pathology underlying the symptoms.

A3: What might the important aetiological factors be?

PREDISPOSING FACTORS

Somatization disorder is more common in patients who have previously had anxiety disorders or depression. In addition, personality factors are likely to be of importance, and she may have a personality disorder.

PRECIPITATING FACTORS

There may be some particular precipitant for this episode such as a current stressor.

MAINTAINING FACTORS

It may also be that there is an apparent gain from her symptoms, such as avoiding an abusive husband, or avoiding work. This may be termed a secondary gain, in that it is not the primary motivation for the symptoms, which is assumed to be subconscious.

A4: What treatment options are available?

LOCATION

Somatization disorders and hypochondriacal disorders should be treated on an outpatient basis.

PHYSICAL

- There is little place for drug treatment in the management of primary hypochondriasis or somatization disorder.
- However, you should always bear in mind the possibility of an atypical depressive episode. A trial of an antidepressant may be considered worthwhile.

PSYCHOSOCIAL

- The following principles should guide initial management:
  - sufficient physical investigation to exclude physical pathology;
  - explain and reassure in the light of negative investigations, while at the same time acknowledging the reality of the symptoms;
  - discuss sensitively the ways in which psychological factors can give rise to physical symptoms, and assess the patient's response to this;
  - follow a firm and consistent policy with respect to further investigations.
- If you wish to embark on a more definitive treatment, you need to consider carefully the patient's response to attempts to construe her symptoms in psychological terms:
  - if she is able to view them in these terms (i.e. she is 'psychologically-minded'), cognitive therapy may be useful;
  - if not, you could consider behavioural therapies This may either take the form of anxiety management techniques or may involve a programme of graded exercise/activity designed to reduce the disability associated with the psychopathology.

A5: What is the prognosis in this case?

- The prognosis of somatization disorder or hypochondriasis is very variable. A good prognosis is suggested by:
  - the presence of comorbid psychiatric illness (because it can be effectively treated);
  - acute and recent onset;
  - normal premorbid personality;
  - good premorbid functioning;
  - good family or social support; and
  - psychological mindedness.
- The prognosis of malingering is dependent on the gain or reason involved.
- The prognosis of factitious disorder is unclear – such patients are very difficult to follow-up.

CASE 7.4 – **Atypical seizures**

A1: What is the likely differential diagnosis?

Preferred diagnosis:

- Dissociative seizures.

Alternative diagnoses:

- Deterioration of epilepsy.
- Malingering.
- Factitious disorder.

A2: What information in the history supports the diagnosis, and what other information would help to confirm it?

- Not all atypical seizures are non-epileptic. It is possible that a stressor such as her husband going away has led to a deterioration in the medical control of her epilepsy. It is common for epileptic seizures to be exacerbated by stress and anxiety. However, non-epileptic seizures are suggested by:
  - a gradual onset;
  - a varied pattern of movements lacking the usual stereotyped nature of epilepsy;
  - a lack of tongue biting, injury and incontinence (though these may occur); and
  - suggestibility (for example, a change in pattern of seizure associated with a comment made during it).
- In addition, you need to consider the patient's history. Non-epileptic seizures may be suggested by a history of:
  - psychiatric disorder;
  - abnormal personality;
  - deliberate self-harm;
  - presence of severe psychosocial stressors.
- Two investigations may be helpful, but neither will always give a firm diagnosis:
  - serum prolactin levels may be raised after a generalized epileptic seizure;
  - electroencephalographic monitoring during an attack may detect seizure activity.
- Non-epileptic seizures may be deliberately and consciously feigned (malingering or factitious disorder), or they may be due to a dissociative disorder (sometimes called a 'conversion disorder'). It is often very difficult to be sure of the degree of consciousness involved, and a simple judgement that it is deliberate or not deliberate is usually not appropriate.
- Straightforward malingering, for financial reward, or to avoid work is usually readily recognizable.
- It is important to note that she may have both epileptic seizures and dissociative seizures. Non-epileptic seizures are more common in people with epilepsy.
- Her relationship with her husband must be assessed, looking in particular for signs of over-dependence.

A3: What might the important aetiological factors be?

PREDISPOSING FACTORS

Dissociative disorders are more likely in people with dependent or anxious personality traits or personality disorder. Such people may also have a history of other anxiety disorders. There is also an association between dissociative seizures and childhood sexual abuse.

PRECIPITATING FACTORS

The imminent departure of her husband may be a source of stress which could exacerbate epilepsy, precipitate a dissociative disorder (in which case her husband staying with her would be a secondary gain), or cause malingering (in which case her husband staying with her would be the primary gain).

MAINTAINING FACTORS

The precipitating factors are likely to be maintaining the disorder.

A4: What treatment options are available?

LOCATION

Somatization disorders and hypochondriacal disorders should be treated on an outpatient basis.

PHYSICAL

There is no pharmacological treatment for dissociation.

PSYCHOLOGICAL

- Once a diagnosis of non-epileptic or dissociative seizures has been made, it is sensible gradually to withdraw anticonvulsants. This should ideally be done in collaboration with the patient, who may need a great deal of reassurance that this is safe. This is particularly difficult if the label of epilepsy is long-standing and if secondary gains are present (such as her dependency on her husband). Her family/carers need to be involved in this cognitive restructuring, enabling her (and them) to accept the change in diagnosis.
- An exploration of the patient's history may yield clues as to a focus for psychological intervention, such as childhood sexual abuse.
- Behavioural anxiety management techniques or problem-solving therapy may also be beneficial if the attacks are associated with anxiety or stress.

SOCIAL

Social interventions should aim to reduce stressors and improve the patient's general life situation.

A5: What is the prognosis in this case?

- The prognosis of dissociative/conversion disorders in general is variable.
- The most important factor is duration before intervention. Conversion symptoms of recent and acute onset have a good prognosis – for example, paralysis may respond to graded exercises or, especially in children, a therapeutic manoeuvre of which spectacular results are promised.
- However, if dissociative states have been present for more than 1 year before reaching psychiatric attention, they are likely to prove resistant to therapy.

♟♟ OSCE counselling cases

OSCE COUNSELLING CASE 7.1

You are asked to see a patient in the accident and emergency department who has taken an overdose of paracetamol. He requires physical treatment for the effects of this in hospital, but is refusing.

A1: What would you do and what advice would you give to the medical staff?

- You need to see the patient and carry out as full an assessment as you can, including trying to access any previous psychiatric notes from your hospital and talking to an informant such as a relative.
- In most cases a patient can be persuaded to accept the treatment if this is dealt with carefully and sensitively at interview. You would need to see him in private in an appropriate room, with a member of nursing or medical staff.
- If he does not consent to the treatment, then he cannot be treated. The only exception to this is if he lacks capacity to give informed consent. In these circumstances, treatment may be given in his best interests, under the common law. A person lacks capacity if they are:
  - unable to make a decision because they are:
    - unable to understand relevant information;
    - unable to retain that information; and/or
    - unable to make a decision based on that information.
  - unable to communicate a decision (e.g. because they are unconscious).
- If the patient has a mental illness then he is liable to detention under the Mental Health Act (MHA) and can be kept in hospital against his will. However, treatment for the physical consequences of his paracetamol overdose is not a treatment for mental disorder and therefore is not covered by the MHA. Even if you were to detain him in hospital because he has depression and you consider him at risk of further self-harm, you still could not enforce the treatment for his paracetamol overdose unless, in addition, he lacks capacity.

A2: Explain how you would carry out an assessment of his risk of self-harm.

You need to think about five areas.

- Assessment of factors known to be associated with suicide:
  - male gender;
  - increasing age;
  - unmarried;
  - chronic or painful illness;
  - unemployed or high-risk occupation (doctor, hotel/bar trade, farmers);
  - social isolation and lack of personal support.
- Previous episodes of self-harm:
  - How often have they occurred before?
  - What has precipitated them previously?
  - Did he write a note or do any other final acts?
  - Was it planned or impulsive?
  - What precautions did he take against discovery?
  - Was it associated with alcohol or drug intoxication?
  - How dangerous did he think the chosen method was?
- Current ideas of suicide:
  - Is he pleased or sorry to be alive?
  - Does he feel hopeless?
  - Can he see a future for himself?

- Are there alternatives to suicide?
- How often does he think about suicide?
- Does he find this distressing or comforting?
- Does he have further plans of how to kill himself?
- What would stop him committing suicide (family, religion, etc.)?
- Does he want help and treatment?
- Psychiatric disorder:
  - The risk of suicide is increased in psychiatric disorder – particularly depression, bipolar affective disorder and schizophrenia – as well as in personality disorder and drug and alcohol misuse.
- Associated risks:
  - Patients who are at risk of suicide may also be at risk of other things such as self-neglect. Impulsive self-harm is also associated with violence to others. Occasionally, a depressed person may have homicidal thoughts in addition to suicidal thoughts.
  - The range of factors that lead to an increased risk of self-harm must be weighed against any protective features to develop an assessment of the overall risk of suicide. This can then be used to formulate a management plan.

REVISION PANEL

- Psychiatric disorders are under-recognized in general healthcare settings.
- Atypical presentations of psychiatric disorder commonly lead to apparently physical presentations.
- A capacity assessment must be specific to the particular decision being taken at the time.
- Assessment of suicide risk is a core skill for all doctors.

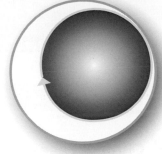

8 Substance misuse

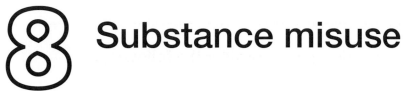

Questions

Clinical cases

For each of the case scenarios given, consider the following:

Q1: What is the likely differential diagnosis?
Q2: What information in the history supports the diagnosis, and what other information would help to confirm it?
Q3: What might the important aetiological factors be?
Q4: What treatment options are available?
Q5: What is the prognosis in this case?

CASE 8.1 – **Heavy drinking**

A 49-year-old bricklayer attended his general practitioner (GP) after experiencing an epileptic seizure. Approximately 5 years previously he had noticed that his hands were shaky in the morning. This would last until lunchtime, when he would drink five or six pints of beer in the pub with his work colleagues. At this point the shakiness would settle and he would feel much better. His daily intake of beer had gradually increased over several years, and he always kept an alcoholic drink beside the bed to have when he woke up to 'steady his nerves for the day ahead'. He had noticed some numbness in both feet, and had brought up some fresh blood while retching. His friends commented that his memory was poor, and he wondered whether his skin might have a yellowish tinge to it.

CASE 8.2 – **Disorientation and hallucinations in a general hospital**

The on-call liaison psychiatrist is asked to see a 43-year-old woman on a surgical ward, as she is distressed and agitated. She was admitted to hospital 48 h previously with abdominal pain, and is known to have had several previous admissions to hospital with similar problems. Her notes record that she had drunk 3 litres of strong cider on the day of admission. She appears extremely shaky, and is disorientated in time and place. She claims to have seen giant spiders climbing up the curtains by her bed.

CASE 8.3 – **Increasing opiate misuse in a young adult with associated problems**

A 23-year-old woman is brought to the GP by her mother, who had been concerned about a gradual deterioration in her daughter's mood and behaviour over the previous 6 months. When caught stealing money from her mother's handbag, the daughter admitted that she was using drugs. She had first smoked cannabis when she was 16, and later experimented with Ecstasy, LSD and amphetamines at weekends. She tried heroin 18 months prior to the consultation, initially smoking it 'on the foil'. Within 6 months she was using it every day, and noticed that she began to experience sweating and generalized muscular aches if she was unable to obtain a daily supply.

OSCE counselling cases

OSCE COUNSELLING CASE 8.1

You are working as a GP when a 37-year-old man comes to see you with a badly bruised arm after a fall. It is 10 a.m., but he smells strongly of alcohol.

Q1: Describe how you would go about assessing any alcohol problem.

Q2: How would you try to improve his motivation to stop drinking?

Q3: What sort of interventions would you consider?

⚷ Key concepts

Problems with alcohol or drugs exist on a spectrum. In the UK, few people drink no alcohol at all, and the majority drink in moderation with few associated problems. However, as consumption levels go beyond about 3 units per day for men and 2 per day for women, physical problems become more likely (see Table 8.1).

Table 8.1 'Units' of alcohol found in common measures of drinks

1 pint of 5 per cent lager	2.8 units
1 pint of 3.4 per cent bitter	1.9 units
Small glass of 13.5 per cent wine (125 mL)	1.7 units
Large glass of 12 per cent wine (250 mL)	3 units
Bottle of wine (12 per cent)	9 units
Bottle of 'alcopop'	1.5 units
Pub measure of 40 per cent vodka (25 mL)	1 unit
Bottle of 40 per cent vodka (700 mL)	28 units

The diagnosis of harmful use is made when an individual has a pattern of substance use that is causing damage to their physical or psychological health. The term 'dependence' has now replaced the vaguer terms 'alcoholic' or 'drug addict', and has a clearly defined meaning. The essential feature of substance dependence is impaired control over drug use, but to have dependence a person must have had three or more of the following in the past year:

- A strong desire or sense of compulsion to take the substance.
- Difficulty in controlling substance-taking behaviour in terms of its onset, termination, or levels of use.
- A physiological withdrawal state when substance use has ceased or been reduced, as evidenced by, for example, the characteristic withdrawal syndrome for alcohol, or use of alcohol with the intention of relieving or avoiding withdrawal symptoms.
- Evidence of tolerance, such that increased doses of the substance are required in order to achieve effects originally produced by lower doses.
- Progressive neglect of alternative pleasures or interests because of substance use, or increased amount of time necessary to obtain or take the substance or to recover from its effects.
- Persisting with substance use despite clear evidence of overtly harmful consequences, such as harm to the liver through excessive alcohol consumption.

Narrowing of the personal repertoire of patterns of alcohol use has also been described as a characteristic feature (e.g. a tendency to drink alcoholic drinks in the same way on weekdays and weekends, regardless of social constraints that determine appropriate drinking behaviour).

The number of units of alcohol in any drink can be calculated using the following formula:

$$\text{Number of units} = \frac{\text{(Volume of drink (in mL)} \times \%ABV)}{1000}$$

where %ABV is the percentage of alcohol by volume.

For example a 500 mL can of strong lager (9 per cent) would contain: $\dfrac{(500 \times 9)}{1000} = 4.5$ units.

MOTIVATION TO CHANGE

The 'stages of change' model (Figure 8.1) developed by Prochaska and DiClemente is useful in the conceptualization and subsequent management of substance misuse problems. Prior to its development, a person's motivation to change their problem behaviour was viewed as 'all or nothing', and those that refused help – or who failed to benefit from it – were considered to have been 'lacking motivation'.

Prochaska and DiClemente studied people who had managed to change their smoking behaviour without formal help. This led to the realization that change is rarely a sudden event, but instead occurs in steps or stages. Furthermore, motivation can be seen as the result of an interaction between the substance user and his or her environment, with the implication that treatment can facilitate an increase in motivation for change. The most common treatment outcome for substance dependence is relapse, with approximately 66 per cent of all research participants returning to drinking by the 90-day follow-up assessment. However, a variety of physical and psychological strategies have now been developed to improve long-term outcomes.

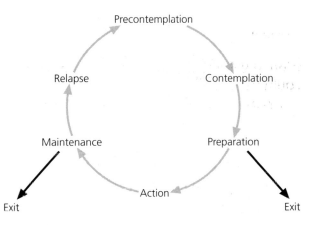

Figure 8.1 The 'stages of change' model.

Answers

Clinical cases

CASE 8.1 – **Heavy drinking**

A1: What is the likely differential diagnosis?

Preferred diagnosis:

- Alcohol dependence.

Alternative diagnoses:

- Epilepsy.
- Amnesic syndrome or dementia.

A2: What information in the history supports the diagnosis, and what other information would help to confirm it?

- This man demonstrates a number of the features of the dependence syndrome, including:
    - increased tolerance to the effects of alcohol;
    - withdrawal symptoms;
    - persistence with drinking, despite negative consequences.
- A detailed history of his pattern and level of alcohol consumption is needed, and this may be facilitated by the use of a drink diary. His experience of withdrawal symptoms must be assessed, including any episodes of delirium tremens. An assessment of any periods of abstinence, their duration and the reason for return to drinking would be useful to plan treatment. A comprehensive assessment of any physical, psychological, social or criminal problems caused by alcohol use is important. A family history of alcohol problems should be obtained, as well as details of any problems that he has experienced with other legal or illegal substances and any previous treatment episodes. Simple self-completion questionnaires such as the Alcohol Use Disorders Identification Test (AUDIT) or the Severity of Alcohol Dependence Questionnaire (SADQ) can help to measure the severity of the problem and plan the appropriate treatment pathway.
- The history of a seizure must be investigated, and memory impairment may suggest that he has developed an amnesic syndrome (Korsakoff's syndrome) or alcoholic dementia.
- Physical examination may show stigmata of chronic liver disease including jaundice, clubbing of the fingers, palmar erythema, spider naevi, gynaecomastia and testicular atrophy. Peripheral neuropathy is another consequence of high alcohol consumption, and it is crucial to exclude the signs of Wernicke's encephalopathy, including ophthalmoplegia, nystagmus and ataxia.
- Simple physical investigations should include:
    - full blood count (FBC) – likely to show a raised mean cell volume and possibly anaemia;
    - urea and electrolytes (U&Es) – possibly deranged sodium or potassium levels secondary to poor diet and vomiting;
    - liver function tests (LFTs) and γ-glutamyl transferase (GGT) – possible evidence of liver damage;
    - blood clotting – markedly abnormal in severe liver disease.

A3: What might the important aetiological factors be?

PREDISPOSING FACTORS

Multiple factors are usually involved in the development of a substance misuse problem in an individual. These may include genetic predisposition, family factors, adverse life events, psychological symptoms, availability and social acceptability of the substance, peer pressure and impoverished educational or work opportunities. It is also clear that depression and anxiety are related to alcohol problems, and substance misuse problems may cause, complicate or be a consequence of mental health problems.

PRECIPITATING FACTORS

In chronic disorders like this it may be difficult to identify specific precipitating or maintaining causes.

MAINTAINING FACTORS

Withdrawal symptoms often necessitate further 'relief' drinking. The consequences of excess alcohol consumption (e.g. marital break-up, unemployment, physical health consequences) may themselves act as stressors that maintain high levels of consumption.

A4: What treatment options are available?

LOCATION

The first stage in any treatment plan for alcohol dependence would be consideration for medically assisted withdrawal from alcohol ('detoxification'). In all but the mildest forms of dependence this will involve the prescription of medication, and as this man has experienced an epileptic seizure, this may have to be in hospital.

PHYSICAL

- A medium- to long-acting benzodiazepine such as chlordiazepoxide (Librium) or diazepam should be initiated at doses sufficient to prevent any significant withdrawal symptoms (usually 20–30 mg chlordiazepoxide, four times daily). This should be withdrawn gradually over 5–7 days.
- Provision of thiamine is essential to prevent the development of Wernicke–Korsakoff syndrome, and this should initially be parenteral.
- Acamprosate and naltrexone are both used to decrease the likelihood of relapse after detoxification and reduce craving for alcohol.
- Disulfiram can be effective when its administration is supervised by someone else as part of a treatment plan.

PSYCHOLOGICAL

- Motivational interviewing is well suited to moving patients towards a firm decision to stop drinking, and aims to mobilize an individual's inherent coping strategies. The technique may incorporate a discussion about the personal costs and benefits of continued drinking balanced against the health and social benefits that would follow a reduction in levels of consumption or abstinence.
- A range of cognitive behavioural techniques may be used at different stages of the problem. It is important to help the patient to set realistic goals and to offer a menu of strategies to help reach these, including self-monitoring, drink refusal skills, assertiveness training, relaxation techniques and the development of alternative coping skills and rewards. Depending on available skills and resources, such interventions may be offered on an individual or a group basis.
- Once withdrawal from alcohol is complete, 'relapse prevention' strategies help to maintain abstinence. The aim is to anticipate and prevent relapses from occurring, and to minimize the negative consequences and maximize learning from the experience if they do.
- Alcoholics Anonymous (AA) may also have much to offer the problem drinker, and this approach can be easily integrated into a treatment programme involving other agencies. AA describes itself as a 'fellowship of men and women who share their experience, strength and hope with each other that

they may solve their common problem and help others to recover from alcoholism'. Self-referral is simple, and the only requirement for membership is a desire to stop drinking. The 'Twelve Steps' and 'Twelve Traditions' of AA help to structure a programme of personal change that can provide life-long support.

SOCIAL

- Alcohol problems can often develop in the context of social stressors such as poor housing, unemployment or interpersonal conflict.
- These problems tend to get worse as alcohol becomes more prominent in a person's life. Whatever the cause, practical attempts to tackle these difficulties can help a person to achieve and maintain treatment goals.

A5: What is the prognosis in this case?

- The chance of relapse is high in the short term, and many people have to attempt detoxification several times before obtaining lasting abstinence.
- Factors that may suggest longer periods of abstinence include:
  - the acceptance of dependence on alcohol;
  - a supportive relationship dependent on abstinence;
  - a negative consequence of continued drinking such as pancreatitis;
  - a source of continued hope;
  - the development of alternative activities to drinking.

CASE 8.2 – **Disorientation and hallucinations in a general hospital**

A1: What is the likely differential diagnosis?

Preferred diagnosis:

- Delirium tremens.

Alternative diagnoses:

- Other causes of delirium.
- Physical causes:
  - liver failure and hepatic encephalopathy;
  - pneumonia;
  - head injury.

A2: What information in the history supports the diagnosis, and what other information would help to confirm it?

- This woman is known to have a history of heavy alcohol consumption, and a detailed alcohol history is likely to highlight the level of her alcohol dependence. However, it is unlikely that it will be possible to obtain much information from her in her current state, so this should be sought from a variety of sources, e.g. nursing staff, relatives, medical notes.
- The features of delirium tremens classically appear at about 48 h after stopping drinking, and include delirium, hallucinations and illusions, tremor, fear, paranoid delusions, restlessness, agitation, and sweating. The disturbance often fluctuates, with the symptoms worsening in the evening. The mental state examination (MSE) may show a fluctuating level of consciousness, poor attention and concentration, delusions, illusions and hallucinations.
- Physical examination may uncover the stigmata of chronic liver disease, and tachycardia and hypertension are common.

- Blood tests may show a variety of abnormalities:
  - U&Es – low potassium;
  - FBC – raised mean cell volume;
  - LFTs – impaired liver function;
  - abnormal blood glucose.

A3: What might the important aetiological factors be?

PREDISPOSING FACTORS

It is unusual for a patient to experience delirium tremens without a history of several years of severe alcohol dependence.

PRECIPITATING FACTORS

Delirium tremens is thought to be directly due to alcohol withdrawal, but it may be precipitated by concurrent trauma or infection.

MAINTAINING FACTORS

These are the same as the precipitating factors.

A4: What treatment options are available?

LOCATION

Delirium tremens is potentially life-threatening, and should always be managed in an inpatient environment.

PHYSICAL

- Treatment is with a drug that is cross-tolerant with alcohol that effectively substitutes for alcohol. Chlordiazepoxide may be given orally in a dosage of up to 400 mg daily in divided doses.
- Antipsychotic medication should be avoided as it can precipitate seizures.
- Fluid and electrolyte balance and blood sugar levels must be carefully monitored
- A patient with delirium tremens is at high risk of developing the Wernicke–Korsakoff syndrome, and should receive regular parenteral doses of a thiamine-containing preparation such as Pabrinex for several days, or until the condition stops improving.
- Seizures usually occur within the first 24 h of admission, but they may also happen during an episode of delirium tremens. They are less likely to occur if the patient has been adequately sedated with benzodiazepines, but there may be an argument for prescribing anticonvulsant medication if the patient is known to have a history of previous withdrawal seizures.

PSYCHOLOGICAL

- Calm consistent nursing in a quiet, well-lit side room.
- Extraneous objects should be removed as they may cause misinterpretations or illusions.

A5: What is the prognosis in this case?

The condition usually lasts for 3–5 days, with gradual resolution. Even with skilled care, death due to cardiovascular collapse, hypothermia or intercurrent infection occurs in about 5 per cent of admissions.

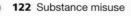

CASE 8.3 – **Increasing opiate misuse in a young adult with associated problems**

A1: What is the likely differential diagnosis?

Preferred diagnosis:

- Opioid dependence syndrome.

Alternative diagnosis:

- Depressive episode.

A2: What information in the history supports the diagnosis, and what other information would help to confirm it?

- An assessment of this young woman's drug problem would include a detailed record of her drug use in the past month, and a full past history. She should be asked about episodes of injection drug use, including whether she has shared injecting equipment and details of high-risk sexual behaviour. Details of any physical, psychological, social or forensic problems relating to her drug use should be sought, as well as an alcohol history. Any previous attempts to stop using drugs may provide useful information for developing a treatment plan, and her strengths, level of social support, and goals for the present treatment contact should be elicited.
- The MSE may reveal symptoms of a comorbid depressive or anxiety disorder, and highlight relevant personality traits.
- Inspection of the skin at the antecubital fossa should be made for signs of injection drug use. A urinary drug screen or saliva test is important to confirm the presence of opioids prior to any medication being prescribed.

A3: What might the important aetiological factors be?

PREDISPOSING FACTORS

Multiple factors are usually involved in the development of a substance misuse problem in an individual. These may include genetic predisposition, family factors, adverse life events, psychological symptoms, availability and social acceptability of the substance, peer pressure and impoverished educational or work opportunities.

PRECIPITATING FACTORS

Peer pressure or curiosity often precipitates initial drug use.

MAINTAINING FACTORS

The predisposing factors are likely to remain present. In addition, comorbid depressive or anxiety disorders or personality disorder may be maintaining drug misuse.

A4: What treatment options are available?

LOCATION

- Treatment will take place in an outpatient setting, either through a community drug treatment team or via the GP with support from specialist services.
- Some residential treatment facilities exist, and admit people for between 3 and 12 months.

PHYSICAL

- The first principle of treatment is 'harm minimization'. Injecting drug misuse carries a significant risk of infection, particularly when equipment is shared or poorly cleaned. Advice about improved injection technique and cleaning of equipment can be effective in reducing this risk, particularly when combined with the provision of clean needles and syringes.
- If this patient wants to stop using opiates, a detoxification may be the logical first treatment step. The opioid withdrawal syndrome is not life-threatening, but is extremely uncomfortable to endure, and provision of medication may assist the person to complete it. Patients using small amounts of heroin may be able to stop abruptly with purely symptomatic support. An explanation of the likely withdrawal side effects and their time course can help to clarify any misunderstandings and improve compliance.
- The GP could prescribe medications such as diazepam (to reduce anxiety, muscle cramps and craving), nitrazepam (to aid sleep) and hyoscine butylbromide (Buscopan; to reduce abdominal smooth muscle spasm) for a period of 7–10 days. Those with dependence on higher doses of heroin or with longer histories of drug use may not be able to tolerate such a simple detoxification process, and will require assessment and management by a specialist drug treatment agency. Lofexidine is another non-opioid option to facilitate detoxification, but causes hypotension so needs some monitoring.
- 'Substitute' prescribing implies the use of a legally prescribed drug such as methadone (a full opioid agonist) or buprenorphine (a partial agonist) instead of an illegal drug of unknown purity and quality. Even if the patient is reluctant, it is vitally important that the doctor tests their urine for evidence of opiate drugs if substitution treatment is to be prescribed. Laboratory tests are detailed and reliable but take some time, whereas 'dipstick' urine screening tests provide an instant result. It is important to recognize the potential for overdose and death if methadone is not initiated at low doses (20–25 mg) and slowly titrated against its effect.
- There is evidence to suggest that the regimens most successful at reducing illicit drug intake are those involving higher daily doses of the substitute drug (approximately 60–120 mg methadone, 12–16 mg buprenorphine), but that the prescription should only occur in conjunction with daily supervision (at least initially) and psychosocial interventions. It may be best to conceptualize the first 3–6 months as a period of stabilization, where attempts are made to develop a 'recovery' plan to mobilize existing resources and tackle any problems. The individual may then choose to withdraw from the medication, or, alternatively, embark on a longer period of 'maintenance' treatment.

PSYCHOLOGICAL

- Someone else has brought this woman for help, and her motivation and commitment to treatment are uncertain.
- Psychological strategies may be directed at motivational enhancement and later relapse prevention.
- Other strategies such as self-monitoring, drug-refusal skills, assertiveness training, relaxation techniques and the development of alternative coping skills and rewards may be important. Mobilizing social network resources and linking to mutual self-help groups (such as Narcotics Anonymous) may help in achieving and sustaining abstinence from illicit drugs.

SOCIAL

- Attempts to help the user improve their supportive relationships, housing and financial situation are likely to considerably improve their motivation to tackle their drug problems.
- Likewise, educational and vocational training will help to fill the time previously spent obtaining and using drugs.
- Many drug users also have criminal convictions pending, and so liaison with probation services can be very important.

A5: What is the prognosis in this case?

- An increasing number of young drug users are presenting to treatment services. It is possible that quick interventions involving detoxification and relapse prevention strategies, combined with social and vocational work, can lead to a good prognosis in this group. Substance use is a relapsing and remitting problem, however, and long-term treatment is common.
- Ultimately, most drug problems seem to 'burn out', with the user making changes to their life that lead to them stopping their drug use. In this respect, if the person does not die from accidental overdose or contract a bloodborne virus such as hepatitis or human immunodeficiency virus (HIV), the prognosis is often better than with alcohol dependence.

⚆⚆ OSCE counselling cases

OSCE COUNSELLING CASE 8.1

You are working as a GP when a 37-year-old man comes to see you with a badly bruised arm after a fall. It is 10 a.m., but he smells strongly of alcohol.

A1: Describe how you would go about assessing any alcohol problem.

- Patients with a range of substance misuse problems may present to the GP, and often the substance misuse problem is not the primary reason for the consultation. Therefore, specific screening and assessment tools exist to enable detection of harmful use of alcohol.
- The CAGE questionnaire is made up of just four questions that can be integrated into a broader enquiry into the patient's health:
  - Have you ever felt you ought to **C**ut down on your drinking?
  - Have people **A**nnoyed you by criticizing your drinking?
  - Have you ever felt **G**uilty about your drinking?
  - Have you ever had a drink first thing in the morning to steady your nerves (an **E**ye opener)?
- A positive answer to two or more or these points suggests that there is a significant problem with alcohol, and a more detailed assessment is necessary. This may take the form of asking the patient to complete a drink diary over the course of a week.

A2: How would you try to improve his motivation to stop drinking?

- **Motivational interviewing** is a style of interviewing particularly suited to helping change problematic behaviours. It involves discussion about the personal costs and benefits of continued drinking when balanced against the health and social benefits that would follow a reduction in levels of consumption or abstinence. It is designed to help those people who are ambivalent about their substance use move towards a firm decision to stop using. In essence, the goal is to have the person talk themselves into deciding to change their behaviour, while emphasizing their right to choose and to accept responsibility for their problems.
- Confronting a person with the need to change often brings about the opposite by precipitating a defensive reaction. For example, telling this man that he drinks too much and ought to stop is likely to just make him annoyed, and the opportunity to help will be lost. Alternatively, an empathic, non-judgemental approach which accepts that he is likely to be ambivalent about changing his drinking behaviour is more likely to engage him in a therapeutic relationship.
- For people in the 'pre-contemplative stage' of change (see Key concepts), providing information can be a useful first step. This may include feeding back the results of his weekly drink diary in the form of units of alcohol per week, but putting this in the context of the national recommended limits (21 units per week for men and 14 units per week for women). Likewise, feedback of mildly abnormal liver function tests may have the effect of raising awareness of the extent of his problem and could start to raise doubts in his mind.
- Asking open-ended questions about his drinking and using reflective listening will start to elicit both positive and negative statements about alcohol. While accepting that there are good things about alcohol, the interviewer tries selectively to reinforce and reflect the bad things that the person themselves suggests, thus accumulating a number of 'self-motivational statements'. These may acknowledge the extent of the problem and indicate a desire for help that can be built upon in further treatment. Another strategy is to contrast the person's previous hopes and aspirations with their current situation, or to ask them how they see themselves in the future. In this case, the man may start to make links between his alcohol use and his failure to achieve promotion at work or other

targets. All the time, the GP should try not to argue or confront the man, but to support his belief that he can change.

A3: What sort of interventions would you consider?

- 'Brief interventions' by GPs to tackle alcohol misuse have been shown to be effective. The simplest of these involves the use of a screening tool followed by:
    - personalized feedback about results of screening/blood tests;
    - offering a 'menu' of alternative coping strategies;
    - information about safe levels of drinking;
    - provision of self-help materials;
    - advice on reducing drinking;
    - ventilation of anxieties and other problems.
- If this man begins to accept the need to change, it is important to work with him to generate realistic goals and to offer a menu of strategies to help reach these. These may include:
    - self-monitoring;
    - setting drinking limits;
    - controlling the rate of drinking;
    - drink-refusal skills;
    - assertiveness training;
    - relaxation training;
    - development of alternative coping skills and rewards;
    - identifying and challenging negative automatic thoughts.
- Once he decides on an appropriate goal, 'relapse prevention' strategies can help support him in maintaining it. The aim is to anticipate and prevent relapses from occurring, but if they do occur then to minimize the negative consequences and maximize learning from the experience. Rather than blaming a patient for difficulties that arise during the course of treatment, emphasis is placed on the specific context and situational factors in which the slip or relapse occurs.
- Participation in a mutual self-help group such as AA may help to build a supportive network, while also reinforcing positive techniques for managing heavy alcohol consumption.

REVISION PANEL

- Substance use problems exist on a spectrum, and are characterized by a strong desire or craving to use a substance, loss of control over use, and resulting medical, psychological and social problems.
- Psychoactive substance use can mimic many other psychiatric disorders, and should always be considered in any differential diagnosis.
- The dependence syndrome has a number of characteristic features including a sense of compulsion to take the substance, difficulty in controlling substance-taking behaviour, a physiological withdrawal state, evidence of tolerance, progressive neglect of alternative interests because of substance use, and persistence with substance use despite clear evidence of harmful consequences.
- Brief interventions aimed at increasing motivation to change substance use are often effective at an early stage of the disorder.
- Treatment strategies may involve medication to reduce the impact of withdrawal symptoms or to reduce the risk of relapse back to regular substance use. However, once dependence is established there is a need to develop new psychological and social strategies for coping with craving and building coping and other skills.
- Mutual self-help, i.e. receiving and providing support from and to other people with addictive problems is an effective strategy in maintaining abstinence over the long term.

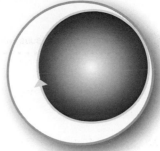

9 Psychiatry and aggression

Questions

Clinical cases

For each of the case scenarios given, consider the following:

Q1: What is the likely differential diagnosis?
Q2: What information in the history supports the diagnosis, and what other information would help to confirm it?
Q3: What might the important aetiological factors be?
Q4: What treatment options are available?
Q5: What is the prognosis in this case?

CASE 9.1 – **Intramarital violence associated with jealousy**

A general practitioner (GP) asks you to see a 52-year-old man. The patient's wife initially contacted the GP because over the past year or so he has gradually become increasingly possessive and jealous. Recently he has begun to accuse her of being unfaithful to him. She says that he never used to be like this, although on very careful enquiry it appears that there have been times in the past when he has been somewhat jealous, although never to this degree. As a result of this jealousy their relationship has steadily deteriorated. Four days ago the man hit his wife during an argument in which he accused her of having an affair. He did not injure her severely, but she is beginning to feel that the only solution is to leave him. He has continued to function reasonably well at work as far as she knows. According to the GP, the man has an erratic employment history and has always been a difficult person. He often tends to take things the wrong way, thinking people are insulting him or making things difficult for him. In fact, he now refuses to see any of the other GPs in the practice because he thinks each one has caused him some problem in the past.

CASE 9.2 – **A man arrested for causing a disturbance in a public place**

You are asked to assess a 32-year-old man who has been arrested by the police for causing a disturbance in the local shopping centre. He was seen attempting to shoplift a leather jacket and, when accosted, became physically aggressive and abusive, making threats to kill the store manager. He has told the police that he is a psychiatric patient and has been an inpatient many times before. He has told them that he should be in hospital because he is depressed. He has been noted to have a number of old superficial cuts on his arm, which appear to have been self-inflicted. He also has a long history of criminal convictions for theft and violent offences. He is apparently intoxicated with alcohol and may be taking other drugs.

CASE 9.3 – **Risk of imminent violence by a psychiatric inpatient with psychosis**

As a core trainee in psychiatry, you are asked to attend the ward to review a male patient who was admitted 2 days ago under Section 3 of the Mental Health Act 1983. He has been complaining of persistent and distressing auditory hallucinations telling him that his parents are going to be killed and that he will be next. He believes that there is some conspiracy against him and his family, led by his former boss at work. He is overactive and sleeping little at night. His speech is fast and difficult to follow, and his mood is changeable, from elation to severe irritability. He has become increasingly aggressive, having smashed a stereo and thrown a coffee mug against the wall. He has been verbally hostile to nurses and other patients. Today, this has escalated further and he is insisting on leaving hospital to go and protect his parents. He has required physical restraint once when he hit out at a member of staff, and is now becoming increasingly agitated again. The nurses feel that further assaults are imminent.

👥 OSCE counselling cases

OSCE COUNSELLING CASE 9.1

A GP asks you to see a patient with a history of admissions to psychiatric hospital, who has been looked after in primary care for some years. The GP is concerned because the patient is complaining of increasing temper and impulsive thoughts of violence. The GP wants you to do a risk assessment.

Q1: Describe how you would go about conducting an assessment of the risk of violence.

⚷ Key concepts

VIOLENCE AND PSYCHIATRIC PATIENTS

The general public tends to overestimate the association between mental disorder and violence. Personality disorder and substance misuse are the diagnostic categories most strongly associated with violence. While there is an increased risk of violence associated with schizophrenia, this is small. Victims of this violence are usually relatives of the patient, and violence towards strangers is rare.

PSYCHIATRIC MORBIDITY IN PRISONER POPULATIONS

Mental disorder is greatly over-represented among prison populations. One influential study reported that only 1 in 10 prisoners do not have some form of mental disorder. Much of this is accounted for by personality disorder and substance misuse diagnoses, but 5–10 per cent of remand prisoners (i.e. charged but not yet sentenced) are psychotic (compared to less than 1 per cent of the general population). The recognition and effective treatment of mental disorders in prison is a major issue for psychiatry, and for the prison service.

THE IMPORTANCE OF ASSESSING THE RISK OF VIOLENCE

The vast majority of psychiatric patients pose no risk to other people. Risk of self-harm and suicide is far more common. Risk of violence may be an issue with respect to particular individuals or with respect to particular types of symptoms (see Table 9.1). In these circumstances, assessment of the risk of violence assumes a greater importance in clinical assessment.

Table 9.1 Individual characteristics and psychiatric symptoms associated with an increased risk of violence

Individual characteristics	Psychiatric symptoms or signs
Dissocial, paranoid, or emotionally unstable personality disorder	Suspiciousness or persecutory thoughts or delusions
Substance misuse	Ideas or delusions of jealousy
Previous history of violence	Delusional misidentification
Impulsiveness	Hostility or anger

Answers

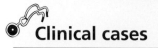 **Clinical cases**

CASE 9.1 – Intramarital violence associated with jealousy

A1: What is the likely differential diagnosis?

Preferred diagnosis:

- Personality disorder, probably paranoid personality disorder.

Alternative diagnoses:

- Alcohol dependence syndrome.
- Persistent delusional disorder.
- Schizophrenia (or other psychotic syndrome).
- Obsessive–compulsive disorder (OCD).
- Depression.

A2: What information in the history supports the diagnosis, and what other information would help to confirm it?

- This is a case of 'morbid jealousy'. Morbid implies that it is pathological. It is pathological because of the distress and problems it is causing for the man and his family. However, morbid jealousy is not a diagnosis. Diagnosis depends on correctly classifying the form of the jealous thoughts and examining the patient for associated symptoms.
- A personality disorder is suggested by the long history of jealousy and the interpersonal problems he has had with respect to his work and his relationships with various GPs. Collecting further, more detailed information about his life from him and his wife, other relatives and perhaps other agencies such as social services or criminal justice agencies would support this diagnosis. You would need to demonstrate that his particular problems have been present persistently since his adolescence, and are so severe as to be significantly different from most people, and cause him personal distress or significant problems in occupational or social functioning.
- Paranoid personality disorder is most commonly associated with morbid jealousy. Such a person will be very sensitive to criticism or rejection and tend to perceive others intentions as hostile or critical even when they are not. These people will persistently hold grudges following such criticism. They tend to be self-important and assertively champion their personal rights. They will be generally suspicious and often jealous and over-protective in intimate relationships.
- The nature of his beliefs must be examined carefully to determine the correct diagnosis:
  - in personality disorder the jealous thoughts will be over-valued ideas;
  - alcohol dependence is also associated with over-valued ideas of jealousy;
  - if the beliefs are obsessions, then OCD may be the diagnosis;
  - depression might present with over-valued ideas of jealousy or delusions of jealousy. You would expect a depressive syndrome to be clearly present;
  - the thoughts might be delusions. In this case, the diagnosis must be a psychotic syndrome. If the patient only has symptoms relating to this jealous theme, does not complain of other psychotic symptoms (such as first rank symptoms of schizophrenia), and the delusions are 'well encapsulated' (he is able to function well at work and continue relatively normal functioning), then the diagnosis is likely to be persistent delusional disorder (delusional morbid jealousy is known as Othello syndrome).

- If he has first rank symptoms as well as delusions of jealousy, then schizophrenia is the likely diagnosis.

A3: What might the important aetiological factors be?

PREDISPOSING FACTORS

Morbid jealousy is associated with alcohol misuse. Other psychological aetiological factors may relate to the man's past history and experience (with respect to his parents, or past sexual relationships) or his particular personality traits (even in the absence of personality disorder).

PRECIPITATING FACTORS

Morbid jealousy is commonly associated with male impotence. Real problems or difficulties in the marital relationship are likely. It is often difficult to disentangle the cause and effect.

MAINTAINING FACTORS

Impotence, alcohol misuse and the marital discord caused by the jealousy are likely maintaining factors.

A4: What treatment options are available?

LOCATION

If there is evidence of a comorbid acute mental illness, such as depression or persistent delusional disorder, then admission to hospital will be likely. If there is no clear evidence of mental illness, you are likely to attempt to manage the case as an outpatient. However, if your risk assessment suggests that the risk of further harm to his wife is likely, then it may be necessary to separate them. A hospital admission would achieve this and may provide a useful temporary resolution to a family in crisis. Particular questions that might be of relevance to the risk assessment include:

- Does he follow his wife when she goes out?
- Does he come home at unexpected times to try and catch her out?
- Has he examined her underwear or clothing?
- Has he questioned her about stains on her clothes, or smells when she comes in?
- Does he scrutinize her mail or set traps in an attempt to catch her out?
- How often do they argue about it?
- How often has he hit her?
- Has he made other specific threats to her?
- Does he think he knows whom she is being unfaithful with? Is this person at risk?

PHYSICAL

Any underlying mental illness should be treated in the usual way.

PSYCHOLOGICAL

- The process of developing a therapeutic relationship and the provision of a safe environment in which he is able to discuss his thoughts and feelings is of great importance to continued risk assessment, and will also help to reduce the risk of violence.
- It may be possible to address his thoughts of jealousy using cognitive therapy. Unfortunately, patients with paranoid personality disorder find it very difficult to form confiding therapeutic relationships, so this may be difficult.

SOCIAL

Paranoid personality disorder is difficult to treat and tends to be persistent. There is also a risk of violence associated with morbid jealousy. It is sometimes said that separation is advisable. In practice you must ensure that his wife is fully informed of the psychiatric aspects of risk and prognosis, so that she can make her own informed decisions. Your must also consider whether anyone else needs to be informed of a risk – someone that he believes his wife is having an affair with, for example.

A5: What is the prognosis in this case?

The prognosis is dependent on the diagnosis.

- If the morbid jealousy is solely a function of a personality disorder, it is likely to be persistent.
- If the patient has a personality disorder but is also suffering from a treatable mental illness, then the prognosis will be better. It is likely that once the mental illness has been treated the thoughts of jealousy will be less intense.
- If there is no evidence of personality disorder and the marriage has previously been stable, the prognosis will be better still.

CASE 9.2 – **A man arrested for causing a disturbance in a public place**

A1: What is the likely differential diagnosis?

Preferred diagnosis:

- Personality disorder, probably dissocial or emotionally unstable.

Alternative diagnoses:

- Mood disorder, either depression or (hypo)mania.
- Psychosis, such as schizophrenia.
- Delirium.
- Malingering.

A2: What information in the history supports the diagnosis, and what other information would help to confirm it?

- The vignette describes multiple, long-standing problems, and this may suggest a personality disorder. The combination of self-harm, criminality and alcohol misuse points to an emotionally unstable or dissocial personality disorder, but to confirm this diagnosis you must collect as much information as possible. Initially, you may be able to access previous psychiatric notes. At interview take a careful developmental history, thinking particularly about his ability to form and maintain interpersonal relationships (with parents, siblings, peers, teachers, employers, lovers), evidence of impulsivity (affective instability, poor performance or behaviour at school, drug and alcohol misuse, previous offending, sexual promiscuity) and evidence of conduct disorder in adolescence.
- Alternatively, or in addition, he says that he feels depressed. A history and mental state examination (MSE) will confirm the presence or absence of a depressive syndrome. Some patients with mania may describe feeling irritable or angry, or may have times when they feel low in mood (often known as dysphoric mania).
- Psychosis would be suggested by a clear description of psychotic symptoms.
- Delirium should be considered in any patient described as intoxicated, as it is an important diagnosis to make promptly.
- Malingering is the intentional feigning of symptoms motivated by external stresses or incentives, which in this case may be the desire to avoid criminal charges.
- Even if he has previously received a diagnosis of personality disorder he may also be experiencing an acute mental illness. It is very important not to assume that people who present in this way have just a personality disorder, as other mental disorders are more common in people with personality disorders.

A3: What might the important aetiological factors be?

PREDISPOSING FACTORS

Dissocial personality disorder is familial, and this is partly genetically determined. So a family history of this or of criminality may be present. It is also associated with a history of emotional or physical abuse in childhood, parental discord, inconsistent parenting, and hyperkinetic disorder in childhood.

PRECIPITATING FACTORS

In patients with a personality disorder the current presentation is likely to have been precipitated by a life event or stressor. This may seem to be a minor event such as an argument with someone or a difficulty at work, but the presence of personality disorder tends to make an individual more susceptible to such stressors.

MAINTAINING FACTORS

Personality disorder is a chronic disorder.

A4: What treatment options are available?

LOCATION

- First of all, you need to know whether the police are going to press charges. The police may be reluctant to charge someone who it considers to be a psychiatric patient. The police should be discouraged from this view, as it is better for the legal process to be continued in parallel to any psychiatric treatment.
- Then, if he is released by the police, continued psychiatric treatment may be carried out in hospital or as an outpatient, as with any other patient.
- If he is kept in custody, further psychiatric assessment and treatment can be arranged. Prisoners may be transferred out of custody to a psychiatric hospital at any stage.

You must consider two main issues to inform any advice you give the police.

- Diagnosis: If the sole diagnosis is personality disorder, it is probably not going to be useful to admit him to a general psychiatric hospital. Such disorders often deteriorate with inpatient treatment. However, if a patient with personality disorder is going through a particular episode of distress, because of some life event or stressor, a short-term crisis admission may be helpful, to remove them from that stress. It may also be an opportunity to help them cope with stresses better in the future. This form of short-term, immediate help is termed 'crisis intervention'. In addition, it should always be remembered that patients with personality disorder are more likely to develop acute mental illnesses, and that the presence of personality disorder may affect the presentation of such an illness. Therefore, always consider whether or not you have truly been able to exclude a depressive episode.
- Risk assessment: A high risk of self-harm may suggest that psychiatric admission is preferable to police custody. If he presents a high risk of harm to others it may be safest for him to remain in custody. Further psychiatric assessment can then be carried out easily, and specialist forensic psychiatric advice may be sought if necessary.

PHYSICAL

- There is little place for medication in the treatment of dissocial personality disorder.
- Sometimes, symptomatic treatment with hypnotics or anxiolytics may be useful, but in such patients the risk of dependence can be high.
- Any comorbid mental illness, such as depression, should be treated vigorously.

PSYCHOLOGICAL

Treatment of dissocial personality disorder is difficult because of the nature of the disorder. However, some patients may be helped by the development of a therapeutic relationship, support in dealing with their problems, and cognitive therapy may be able to examine and modify his habitual ways of thinking about himself and his relationship.

SOCIAL

Help with finances, housing, employment and support with respect to criminal charges may occasionally be useful.

A5: What is the prognosis in this case?

His personality disorder will be long-standing. However, if his current presentation is caused by an acute crisis, then it may be possible to support him through this until he feels more stable. He will nonetheless remain liable to further such episodes in the future.

CASE 9.3 – Risk of imminent violence by a psychiatric inpatient with psychosis

A1: What is the likely differential diagnosis?

Preferred diagnosis:

- Schizoaffective disorder, manic type.

Alternative diagnoses:

- Schizophrenia.
- Manic episode.
- Delirium.
- Drug or alcohol misuse.

A2: What information in the history supports the diagnosis, and what other information would help to confirm it?

- The persistent auditory hallucinations and persecutory delusions indicate that he is psychotic. His overactivity, labile mood, poor sleep and rapid speech may suggest that he fulfils diagnostic criteria for mania as well as schizophrenia, and that therefore schizoaffective disorder, manic type is an appropriate diagnosis.
- Alternatively, you may decide that his psychosis is paramount and the mood element is not sufficiently prominent to justify schizoaffective disorder as a diagnosis. Then schizophrenia would be the most appropriate diagnosis.
- In a manic episode, you would expect the mood disorder to have preceded the development of psychosis.
- There is nothing to suggest delirium, but in any acute and florid presentation it should be considered and excluded.
- His risk of violence appears to be directly related to his psychotic symptoms. However, it may be that he has a history of violence while not unwell. If so, this would suggest that other factors such as personality disorder, drug or alcohol misuse may be important.
- The association of drug and alcohol misuse with violence occurs across all psychiatric diagnoses. Intoxication may make violence more likely in a patient who is also psychotic.

A3: What might the important aetiological factors be?

PREDISPOSING FACTORS

Factors associated with violence may be important, such as previous violence, personality disorder, substance misuse and impulsivity.

PRECIPITATING FACTORS

His psychotic symptoms seem to have precipitated his current violence. Among inpatients, violence is particularly likely when manic symptoms and psychosis coexist. Drug or alcohol intoxication may be another important precipitant.

MAINTAINING FACTORS

Ongoing psychosis, intoxication or mood disorder are likely to maintain his risk of violence. There may be other maintaining factors external to the patient, related to the ward environment or the nature of other patients on the ward.

A4: What treatment options are available?

LOCATION

- If the risk of violence seems imminent, you may consider requisitioning additional nursing staff from other wards and attempting to separate the patient from other patients, in order to ensure a safe and controlled environment. This must be done sensitively to ensure that the patient is not further angered.
- It may be necessary to move him to a psychiatric intensive care unit. This would provide improved physical security such as locks on the doors, as well as increased numbers of staff trained to deal with physical aggression.

PSYCHOLOGICAL

- The first step is to see the patient, attempt to conduct a MSE and gain an empathic understanding of his concerns and distress.
- You should allow the patient as much time as necessary to air his preoccupations and concerns. If a rapport can be established, this may help to defuse the situation and calm the patient down.
- You also need to consider your own safety. You should not see him alone, and nursing staff should always be aware of your location.

PHYSICAL

- The pharmacological management of imminent violence is sometimes known as 'rapid tranquillization'.
- Oral drugs should always be offered first. In some cases, oral sedatives are absorbed as quickly and more reliably than the equivalent intramuscular (i.m.) preparation. Intravenous (i.v.) sedation is rarely required. Two classes of drugs may be used:
  - benzodiazepines – these are the safest, as overdose is unlikely and may be reversed using a benzodiazepine antagonist (flumazenil);
  - sedative antipsychotics (haloperidol and olanzapine may be given i.m.) – these have a possible advantage in patients with psychosis, although the antipsychotic effect is not immediate.
- The two classes are often used together. A common combination would be 5–10 mg haloperidol and 1–2 mg lorazepam (depending on the age and physical state of the patient). These drugs are chosen because of their relatively short half-lives.
- The doses may be repeated at 30-min intervals until a satisfactory response is achieved.
- In patients with cardiac disease, benzodiazepines should be used alone. In patients with compromised respiratory function, benzodiazepines should be avoided.

- A further option is the short-acting depot zuclopenthixol acetate. This is an i.m. antipsychotic preparation that produces peak levels after 24–36 h and is effective for 72 h. This is most useful for managing an ongoing but short-term risk of violence as it takes several hours to reach peak levels. It should not be given to patients who have not previously been exposed to antipsychotics, or to those who are actively struggling in physical restraint.
- Subsequently, the patient must be carefully monitored – respiratory rate (benzodiazepine toxicity), blood pressure, heart rate, presence of extrapyramidal side effects (antipsychotics) and level of consciousness/aggression.
- Continued attempts should be made to reassure the patient, calm him down verbally, and build a therapeutic relationship.

A5: What is the prognosis in this case?

- The short-term prognosis of violence or aggression occurring as a consequence of severe mental illness is good, and it is likely to respond quickly to the management outlined above.
- The ongoing risk of violence will need to be considered once the patient is well. It may be that the risk of violence is entirely dependent on his mental health, and is unlikely to reoccur if he remains well.
- Alternatively, other factors may come to light on recovery, such as personality disorder, drug or alcohol misuse, or a long history of violence and aggression. This points to a high risk of further violence, even in the absence of a relapse of his mental illness.

⛐ OSCE counselling cases

OSCE COUNSELLING CASE 9.1

A GP asks you to see a patient with a history of admissions to psychiatric hospital, who has been looked after in primary care for some years. The GP is concerned because the patient is complaining of increasing temper and impulsive thoughts of violence. The GP wants you to do a risk assessment.

A1: Describe how you would go about conducting an assessment of the risk of violence.

- First of all, you need to consider where it is safe to see the patient. In practice, you are likely to see him in the outpatient department. You need to consider whether you should have someone else with you, and if not you should ensure that other staff know your location. You might consider keeping a personal alarm with you during the interview.
- Clarify issues with the GP, who will be able to give further useful information about the patient.
- As well as seeing the patient you need to try to collect further information from independent sources. You will need the patient's permission to do this. For example, you may be able to interview a wife or partner, or there may be police records or social services records to see. You would also need to look at his previous psychiatric notes.

You need to consider five areas.

- Assessment of factors known to be associated with violence:
  - previous violence is the strongest predictor of future violence, particularly if violence occurred at a young age;
  - male gender;
  - personality disorder more than mental illness;
  - drug and alcohol misuse;
  - childhood physical abuse;
  - parental substance misuse or criminal history;
  - poor adjustment at school;
  - employment problems;
  - previous failure of supervision by psychiatric services, criminal justice agencies, etc.
- Consideration of previous episodes of violence:
  - frequency – the more often it has occurred in the past, the more likely it is to occur again;
  - victims – spouse, random strangers, carers, health professionals;
  - severity;
  - Have weapons been used?
  - What injuries were caused or could have been caused?
  - range of circumstances:
    - Only in association with alcohol/drug intoxication?
    - Impulsive or premeditated?
    - Only during previous episodes of mental illness?
    - Precipitants of previous violence?
- Current thoughts or ideas about violence:
  - What is his mood like? How angry is he? Does he feel humiliated or vengeful?
  - Is he hostile, irritable or aggressive during the interview?
  - What are his views on violence? Does he feel it is sometimes justified?
  - Has he had any thoughts or impulses to hurt someone? What about when he is really angry or fed-up? If so who?

- Has he made any plans to commit violence?
- Does he have any weapons available that he would use?
- The presence of psychiatric disorder:
  - What is the diagnosis and what does the patient think of this?
  - Does he have any insight?
  - Are you able to discuss with him the ways in which mental illness may have affected his thinking?
  - Does he think that he requires treatment?
  - Is he willing or able to work collaboratively with a psychiatric team?
- The presence of associated risks:
  - Patients who are at risk of violence may also be at risk of other things such as self-neglect and suicide. Impulsive violence is strongly associated with suicide.

REVISION PANEL

- Most patients with mental disorder pose no increased risk of violence to other people.
- There is a small increased risk of violence associated with schizophrenia and psychosis, but personality disorder and substance misuse are the disorders with the strongest association.
- Certain key symptoms may herald a possible increased risk. Clinicians must be aware of these and carry out a further assessment of risk of violence when they are present.

Index

Notes
Pages numbers in **bold** denote tables or boxes
Pages numbers in *italics* denote figures